MW01291525

QUANTUM
MITOCHONDRIAL
NUTRITION

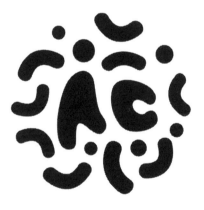

DR. AYSEGUL CORUHLU

About the Author

Dr. Aysegul Coruhlu was born July 4, 1969. She completed her secondary education in Izmir and graduated from the Istanbul Faculty of Medicine in 1994. While specializing in biochemistry at Sisli Etfal Hospital, she studied for her master's program in biomedical engineering at Bosphorus University.

Dr. Coruhlu began to work as a biochemist at the American Hospital in 2000. She later became the head of the Intermed Polyclinic Laboratory. Dr. Coruhlu also received training at the American Anti-Aging Academy.

She was one of the first to implement advanced anti-aging approaches such as antioxidant tests, tests measuring the speed of aging, hormone and genetic tests, the alkaline diet, prescribing tailor-made vitamin and mineral boosts, and intravenous antioxidant applications.

Dr. Coruhlu has focused on preserving health at the cell level.

The author has published two more books, *Alkali Diyet* ("The Alkaline Diet") and *Tokuz ama Aç•z* ("We are Full yet Hungry").

Contents

Foreword

Why do we consider it normal to get ill?
Why do we consider aging normal?

Have you ever thought about these questions? A simple answer may be the following: **because we aren't robots**. We, human beings, are biological creatures. We have a very complex biological structure. Our biology sets the rules.

- *So, in simple terms, we get ill if our biology breaks down.*
- *We age as our biology wears down over the years.*
- *And death is inescapable.*

This answer is correct. But not quite "shrewd" enough; because even though we are biological creatures, we do not sufficiently question whether our daily lifestyles suit our biology.

- Is the packaged and processed food we eat suitable for our biology?
- Is the water we drink, the air we breathe and the electromagnetic pollution we are exposed to suitable for our biology?
- Are the therapies, the antibiotics, and the chemotherapy used when we get ill suitable for our biology?
- Are the houses we live in and the buildings we work in suitable for our biology?

How, despite all medical advances, do we explain the rise in illnesses? Why do you think illnesses have increased? Would you like to take a look at the list below?

In children:

- obesity
- attention deficit disorder (ADD)
- autism

In the young:

- polycystic ovary syndrome (POS)
- acne
- excess body and facial hair
- gynecomastia
- insulin resistance in the under-20-year-olds

In adults:

- thyroid disorders

- incessant allergies

- gastrointestinal disorders

- flatulence

- indigestion

- constipation

- irritable bowel syndrome (IBS)

- infertility

- Psychological problems that are becoming widespread among all ages:

- depression

- panic attacks

- obsessions

- sleep disorders

And of course, there are **Alzheimer's, brain fog, and cancer**.

Calculating the probabilities, how long will it take for these illnesses to catch up with us? Perhaps our heads are so deep in the sand that we believe we'll not figure in that equation. Or, perhaps we have every confidence in medicine.

True, a lot of medical research is individually

carried out on diseases, and treatments are discovered. But so far, the issue has never been examined from the perspective of biological rules. Since we can all agree that we are not mechanical robots but instead biological creatures, we should question which biological rule has been broken to cause all these illnesses.

Let me explain. We are making a mistake in the choice of energy that ensures our biological vitality. In other words, we are not eating in a way that is appropriate for the biology of our **mitochondria**—our source of life, our energy engines.

The thousands of mitochondria in each of our cells are there only for us to produce energy. Altogether they number trillions, and we are dependent on them.

- Even a strand of our hair cannot grow without the energy from mitochondria.
- Our aging cells cannot be renewed without the energy produced by mitochondria.
- We will not recover from diseases if mitochondria do not produce energy.

We are dependent on that energy for something as simple as blinking an eye and something as vital as our immune system intercepting a cancer cell. All our life functions are dependent on that energy. We must secure that energy. **And what's more, we must do this for every second of twenty-four hours a day.** We must do whatever it takes for our mitochondria to produce that energy for us. We must give whatever source of energy they choose as fuel to these energy engines. **Otherwise, we shall die.**

Our afflictions in illness and cures in treatment are the same for all of us: choosing the most appropriate fuel for our mitochondrial engine, so that it may produce the best energy.

That is our fundamental task. That is our prime concern. The best fuel is the most appropriate one (nothing more) for our mitochondria's biology, our mitochondria's **quantum biology**. Classical biology is now inadequate in explaining the complex energy production in mitochondria. **The new biology is quantum biology.**

If we want to stay alive for many years and live a healthy life, we cannot go against the unequivocal principles of biology. We receive energy that supplies our vitality according to quantum biological principles of mitochondria. In other words, we must abide by the rules of quantum biology.

Biology is unforgiving.

And so, here we have the theme of this book:

Human beings produce energy according to quantum principles.

Therefore, human beings need to eat what is consistent with quantum biology.

Human beings must eat quantum.

Introduction:

From the Elixir of Immortality to Nanorobots

It can be said that throughout history, nearly every human being—whatever their creed, race, culture, and outlook on life may be—has wished not to die and has expressed the desire for immortality in various ways: through symbols, myths, epics, and metaphors. Hence, the pursuit of immortality is among the oldest and most deep-rooted quests in human history.

Elixirs of Immortality

A popular narrative in Anatolia relates that Lokman Hekim[i] found **ab-• hayat** *(elixir of immortality)* but dropped it into the water crossing a bridge. We have a saying referring to immortality, "*If he [Lokman Hekim] hadn't lost the elixir to life, humankind would have been immortal and lived forever in this world.*"

If we were to look at medieval Europe, we would

see that there was no distinction between science and sorcery. For instance, a rumour spread that the amateur chemist Nicolas Flamel discovered the *Elixir of Life* during his alchemy experiments. Accordingly, anyone who drank this magic potion became immortal. Thus, the idea of an elixir for immortality began to fascinate other scientists as well, and many of them including Isaac Newton tried to copy Flamel's methods.

In 1513, the Spanish explorer Juan Ponce de León set out to find the source of the legendary *Fountain of Youth*. There was a rumour that the water from the fountain rejuvenated people, and those who drank from it defied death. Queen Isabel and King Ferdinand were among the people who believed it, and they instructed famous explorers in finding the fountain.

Modern Times: Calorie Restriction.

In modern times, the secret of a long life became a topic of scientific research. In a study by Cornell University in 1934, it was observed that diet **extended the lifetime of mice**. While one group of mice was given a normal diet, another group was given a **calorie restricted** diet. The second group of mice lived twice as long as the first group. The same experiment was subsequently carried out with fruit flies, primates, and humans.

Freeze–Wait–Reanimate

In 1967, psychology professor James Bedford died of

cancer. Before he died, he wanted to have his body frozen and have it wait to be thawed sometime in the future. At the time, there was a group of scientists who were researching this subject. They used liquid nitrogen to freeze Bedford's body and placed him in a metal tank. Today, Bedford is still inside that tank. Maybe one day we will discover immortality, and then we will have to reanimate him. **James Bedford was the first person in the history of man to have himself frozen to be thawed at a later point in time**. After him, 230 other people have had themselves frozen; they are now waiting in tanks full of liquid nitrogen to be thawed at a later date.

Charging Your Mind

In 1971, George M. Martin, an expert in geriatric problems, suggested a way to continue living beyond our bodies: **to upload our minds to computers**. Martin said that if computer systems continue to develop very fast, they will work out all the mechanisms of the brain and find a way to convey them to a computer. Today, this idea has become a field in which many scientists are working. The futurist Ray Kurzweil is among those who support similar research.

Medical Nanorobots

By 1986, Eric Drexler, an expert in nanotechnology, stated that in the future we would begin to treat illnesses using microscopic robots that could move inside the human body. Today, the first examples of these nanorobots are already being produced. **One day, nanorobots will also be able to tackle some of the illnesses that are closely associated with aging, such as heart disease, diabetes, or Alzheimer's.**

Genetic engineering, stem cell treatments, 3D replacement organ printing, and new studies for which we haven't even got a name yet are all results of human beings striving for a long and healthy life.

So, in other words, since the times of Lokman Hekim, we have always been galvanized by the same fundamental sentiment: to find the secret to achieve the longest life possible.

Where is that secret then?

Do You Have 140 Birthday Candles?

Well, I too began to pursue this secret. As a doctor and clinical biochemist of twenty-five years, I have always been working at the root of health issues. In order to discover the secret, I studied the smallest components of the body which form the whole: the cells. When it concerned heart diseases, I learned about the biochemical functions of heart cells; when it was brain diseases, I learned about those of brain cells. This made me a good cell-doctor.

Just as I thought I had learned all there was to know

about cells, I discovered something when I was studying for my biomedical master's degree: it was not only biology and chemistry that was involved in the subject of the working of cells, but it was also physics. At the time, it took me somewhat by surprise. But, I was truly amazed when a few years ago I learned **that quantum biology** was also a part of this process.

The human being is a very superior organism. **We need help from other sciences to search for the secret that ensures that this complicated organism always remains healthy and long-lived**. Classical science, which we have been relying on for years, is no longer sufficient when it comes to explaining the superior human being. This is why scientists from different branches must work together to find the answer. Being a doctor alone does not reveal the secret of this masterpiece of an organism. We need help.

On the other hand, I seem to have caught a glimpse of the secret.

The secret is hidden in our most fundamental building blocks: **the cells**. As you read this book, you will learn about just one cell in our complex organism. It is in the activity in that cell that this very important but quite simple secret will be revealed. You, the readers of this book, will learn about this secret before many health care professionals who have failed to notice it.

But why has it taken this long to discover it? Why is it that in all this time we haven't observed the secret between falling ill and being healthy? Why is it that we have never realized that whatever the name of the illness may be, recovery is found in the revelation of the same secret?

Engine and Fuel

The simplest way to explain the secret is as follows: the relationship between the quality of the gasoline you put in your car and its performance is also true for your body. **The secret is in how the *engine* works and in the choice of the most appropriate fuel for it.**

This might seem very simplistic to you right now. However, the purpose of writing this book is to reduce the contrast between illness and health to one single fundamental secret and generic solution. This is not an exaggerated statement. It reflects the basic truth. The most essential fact is the biological needs of our cells. If we can meet the biological needs of our cells, they will reward us.

The reward is a very long and very healthy life. For this we need to answer only two questions:

1. Where is the *engine* of our body?
2. What is the *correct fuel* for this engine?

Let us start with the answer to the first question. Our engines are our ***mitochondria***. This name that we still remember from our high school days refer to the small organelles in the cell that produce energy. You don't need to remember any more than that at the moment; we will be discussing them throughout the book. A large component of the big secret is hidden in our mitochondria.

So, what is our fuel? Now hang on to your hat! The correct answer is the **sun**. Yes, the sun as we know it.

Part of the secret is hidden in the mitochondria, and part is hidden in the sun. We, in fact, extract fuel from the sun—the inexhaustible, mighty source of energy. So, why shouldn't we possess an inexhaustible potency just like the sun? Why only settle for not being ill; why should we not remain young throughout a long lifetime? Why shouldn't we be the luckiest civilisation out of all those that throughout history have searched for the secret of eternal youth? My personal view is that this is a reasonable ambition. **It is not a dream**.

Now, instead of a book full of promises, quite to the contrary, you are going to read a book full of data based on pure science with down-to-earth realism, including cell biochemistry and the quantum physics of atoms.

If you are keen to learn the secret of a long and healthy life, I wish you a happy 140th birthday in advance!

---

[i]The master of all physicians and healers according to centuries-old Turkish legend. It is believed that he had knowledge about the uses of every flower and herb for healing diseases.

How Should You Use This Book?

My devoted followers will immediately remember my two previous books:

1. **Alkali Diyet** *(The Alkaline Diet)*

   A guidebook to preserving the body's pH balance for a long and healthy life.

2. **Tokuz Ama Aç⋅z** *(We Are Full Yet Hungry)*

   An alkaline diet fills your cells, not your stomach.

In the first book, I explained the biochemical logic of nutrition in my capacity as both a doctor and a biochemist. What did we learn from that book? Let's take a quick look.

- ✓ The close relationship between the acid-alkaline balance in our body fluids and the food we eat.

- ✓ Nourishment isn't only about counting calories.

- ✓ The benefits and damage caused by foodstuffs after they have been digested and absorbed into the bloodstream.

The Alkaline Diet shows us that we can turn healthy eating into a lifestyle. It teaches us to use our power in choosing food to our own advantage not only to lose weight but to protect ourselves from illnesses. In short, the first book explains nutrition through simple human biochemistry. And this is only the **introduction** to that which concerns nutrition.

In my second book *We Are Full Yet Hungry*, however, we learn the following:

✓ The concept of nutrition on the cellular level

✓ What is nutrition for our stomach, and what is nutrition for our cells in our choice of food.

✓ The only food our cells require is genuine nutrition, not what modern industry imposes.

✓ The damage caused inside a cell by unwanted food is the common cause of all illnesses.

✓ * For one of our organs to get ill, first that organ's cells must get ill.

✓ Our daily choice of nutrition is the biggest reason for diseases that could afflict us today, seven, or seventy years later.

✓ How to take precautions

We Are Full Yet Hungry is the **development** section on nutrition.

The purpose of reading the book you are now holding in your hands must be to want more than you what get from health books. In any case, your demands from health books should not be modest goals such as losing weight. You must have picked up this book for the following reasons:

- ✓ To not get ill

- ✓ To have perfect health

- ✓ To learn the secrets necessary for a very long life

- ✓ To achieve supreme physical and mental performance

- ✓ To properly master the difference between vitality and lethargy and understand how to increase your vitality

- ✓ To maximize your mental, physical, and sexual capacity

- ✓ To biologically resolve the secret of being a supreme human being

- ✓ To discover how to enable expansion of your biology and your awareness

✓ To understand that learning classical biology and biochemistry is not enough to fundamentally absorb and do all of this, and that you now need to take a step towards the world of quantum—the last point that science has reached.

Now let us take a closer look at ourselves from the world of **quantum** biology. Be ready to take a leap of realization.

This book is the section containing the CONCLUSION on nutrition.

This book is the END-POINT reached by science on nutrition.

Chapter I:

Quantum Biology: A New Biology

Quantum physics has long since entered our lives as a continuation of Newtonian physics. The term **"quantum biology,"** however, was a concept formed when the classical sciences—with which we formerly made do in understanding the world—became inadequate in explaining the biological phenomena, and the subatomic world entered our biological structure.

- *Quantum biology can answer a great many questions we have been curious about but have remained unanswered.*

- *Quantum biology combines physics and biology in the subatomic world.*

Atom: The Essence of Everything

Everything that is **"matter"** in the world and universe

results from the same foundation: atoms. We ourselves, plants, rocks, insects, the air, meteors… everything is formed from atoms. Cells, our minutest units, are also formed from atoms.

In simple terms, the atom is as such: a nucleus, and subatomic particles called **protons** and **neutrons** in the nucleus, with **electrons** scattered like a cloud in the gravitational field around the nucleus but at varying distances from it. You see, the essence of everything is such a tiny structure.

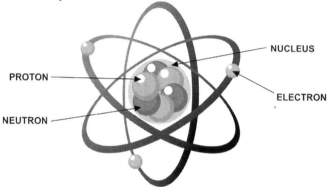

Figure 1: The atom and subatomic particles

Protons are positively (+) charged and electrons are negatively (-) charged. Positive and negative attract each other. If it weren't for this attraction, we could not exist as matter, and we would disintegrate in space. In stable atoms, the number of protons is equal to the number of electrons. Attraction between positive and negative is also equal. So, the attractions are balanced. In unstable atoms, however, the positive and negative numbers are not equal, and this inequality is undesirable. Throughout this book, we will be discussing these atoms.

We like stable atoms; they stay just as they are and do not harm anyone. **But for life on earth to exist, they have to come together to meet each other in order for the chemical reactions of atoms to generate other matter.** Just as it is in water, $H \bullet O$ is two hydrogen atoms and one oxygen atom bonding together.

Therefore, the formation of molecules, from atoms that have bonded together, and the formation of matter from molecules ultimately form us. **The basis of matter is atoms that have bonded together.** However, there is not only matter in the universe.

The Universe Is a Soup of Energy

The whole universe is formed of energy. In fact, matter is compressed energy. The most basic knowledge Einstein has taught us is that matter and energy are the same thing. They are interchangeable. If an atom is matter, it can also be converted into energy.

Foods too consist of atoms. When we eat these substances, they transform into energy inside us.

That is the purpose of nutrition: taking the latent energy in food that is transformed into matter and using it.

Well, if food is matter, isn't it also formed from energy? If we get energy from food and live, from where did food get the energy to become matter in the first place? In other words, what is the first source from which we indirectly get our energy?

The Answer Is Simple: The Sun!

Are We Eating the Sun? We owe our life to the sun. Not only humans but all living creatures owe their lives to the sun. Sunlight is the basic energy source of life. **Light is a quantum phenomenon**. Light is not something straight and continuous; it spreads in waves. The unit of sunlight is a *photon*.

When sunlight, or photons reach the earth, the plants on the earth open their leaves and wait for it. The vitality of plants occurs through photosynthesis, by which the photons from the sun are converted into energy. Photosynthesis, which we all know about, is an important phenomenon that should not remain solely in secondary school biology textbooks. In fact, **photosynthesis is a remarkable quantum biological process.**

Photosynthesis: The First Link in the Food Chain

Clusters of photons are absorbed by energy factories called *chloroplast,* which are found on the leaves of the plant. The plant absorbs and retains the light with *chlorophyll* found in chloroplast. In short, **the plant eats light.**

The plant produces its own energy by taking the

light from the sun, carbon dioxide from the air, and water from the soil. In the plant's energy factories known as chloroplast, these raw materials are converted into energy. Although the plant uses some of this energy to grow and repair itself, it mostly stores it all.

The stalks and fruit of plants are sunlight stored as energy. Through quantum principles, the plant uses sunlight to store the energy it obtains in the **electrons** of the chemical bonds that form these structures.

To sum up briefly:

Sunlight reaches the plants.

↓

The plants "eat" the sun through photosynthesis.

↓

Light turns into energy with carbon dioxide and water in the chloroplast, the plant's battery.

↓

Energy collects in electrons in the plant's stalk, leaves, seeds, and fruit.

↓

When we eat plants, we take our place in the sequence of quantum biological phenomena.

When we eat plants, we transform the sunlight stored by the plant once more into energy. **We convert the materialized sunlight once again into energy. And this is what we call "nutrition."**

Nutrition basically means the transference of sunlight to us through plants. We eat plants as food. We digest them and obtain energy from them in our mitochondria, our energy engines.

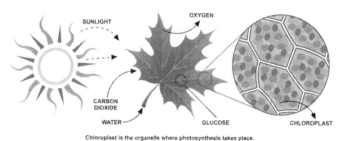

Chloroplast is the organelle where photosynthesis takes place.

Figure. 2: Photosynthesis

We Are Battery-Operated Dolls: Mitochondria and Energy

As the most important tiny organ in the whole body, mitochondria deserve special interest. Our mitochondria give us our energy, which provides us with all our vitality. **There are about forty trillion cells in our body, and each one contains a different number of mitochondria.** There are between 2,500 and 10,000 mitochondria in the cells of organs like the muscles, heart, and brain—which need a lot of energy—and an average number of 500 mitochondria in other cells.

Incredible numbers emerge if we multiply the number of our mitochondria with the number of cells in our body. The reason I am giving so much numerical data is to explain the importance of the topic of energy production in these tiny, rarely mentioned batteries of ours called mitochondria and to justify how seriously it needs to be taken.

Mitochondria should be taken very seriously. Furthermore, a subject that needs to be taken even more seriously is the type of food with which the mitochondria produce better energy and generate less waste as a result of this energy metabolism. **When talking about recipes, calories, diet and slimming, we must redetermine the importance of the tons of health information out there and focus on the increase of energy production in the mitochondria.**

- Mitochondria descend only from the maternal line!

- There are a great many mitochondria in the mother's egg.

- Broadly speaking over 100,000!!!

- In sperm, however, there are almost no mitochondria.

We can say that in the job of obtaining energy – that is in the provision of our battery – our father has little function.

Information on Nutrition of the Future:

✓ nutrition to make the mitochondria healthier

✓ nutrition to make the mitochondria produce more energy

✓ nutrition to make the mitochondria generate less waste

✓ nutrition to make the mitochondria function longer

Future information on nutrition should consist of these suggestions. This is because the faults in the performance of the mitochondria do not manifest themselves merely as energy production faults. Faults make their presence known sometime later as diseases.

Every conceivable disease occurs from the fact that the millions of mitochondria established in the cells in the tissues of that organ have not produced enough energy. If energy is insufficient, then that organ cannot function well. Symptoms caused by a badly functioning organ will take you to that organ's physician, and you will be given a diagnosis.

However, the real diagnosis should be this: your mitochondria are sick!

In that case, in order to increase our respect for our mitochondria, we should continue to learn about their function in energy production, which determines our place between life and death.

Mitochondria are the fireplaces where food is burnt with oxygen.

To produce energy in mitochondria there are two basic requirements: fuel, and oxygen for the fuel to burn. **Burning the food with oxygen occurs only in the mitochondria**. The importance of aerobic respiration is its contribution to our evolution. **We have been able to evolve because of our mitochondria's capacity to produce high energy using oxygen. For millions of years, we have used high energy we have obtained to form a more developed brain.**

Our acquisition of high energy comes from food being burnt with oxygen in the mitochondria. Without oxygen, burning is impossible. The burning of our food inside us is no different from coal burning in a fireplace. Coal keeps energy inside it. When it burns with oxygen, this energy emerges. The coal coming from food (the latent energy in food) is transformed into energy by burning (aerobic respiration) in the mitochondrial fireplace. The energy formed is stored as **Adenosine Triphosphate (ATP)**—energy's currency. This money is changed and spent as needed.

ATP: The Body's Currency

Let us go back to our chemistry classes from school and remember the following: ATP is our energy unit. We eat food in order to ultimately obtain ATP. This is because ATP is the main fuel unit the cells and body use for energy. Everything, including repair, reproduction, and the growth of our hair takes place by consuming ATP.

- Ten million molecules of ATP energy are obtained per second from the mitochondria in a single cell.
- The total ATP amount in our 40 trillion cells corresponds to 60-100 kg of ATP a day.
- We produce ATP energy equal to almost our own weight, and we do this every day.

In fact, there are only 60 grams of ATP in the body that are on standby. This means that after all the ATP reserves are made, they are spent and replenished twice a minute for our daily energy requirement.

In other words, we are in fact charged every half a minute!

The situation when this does not occur is called death. Death is the name of the state when ATP is unobtainable in the body. What prevents us from dying are our energy batteries—the mitochondria.

Thankfully we have a lot of batteries: there are one quadrillion mitochondria in forty trillion cells.

The single secret of longevity is in the mitochondrial membrane.

*The mitochondrial **matrix** is surrounded by a membrane.* In fact, the whole story is in the matrix as this membrane provides our vitality, and it must always be healthy. This is because it is only here that we can produce the **high energy** we mentioned.

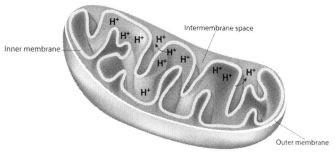

Figure 3: Mitochondrion

Where energy is produced in the cell is a matter which has a great influence on health. There are two separate energy productions in the cell: in one, energy is produced in the mitochondria; and in the other, outside them. From now on, I shall call the energy produced in the mitochondrial matrix ***Plan A high energy production*** and the energy produced outside the mitochondrion (in the part we call the **cell** cytoplasm) ***Plan B low energy production.***

Plan A energy production occurs in the mitochondrial matrix. High energy is obtained there. In other words, much ATP is formed. The mitochondrial matrix is the place where the oxygen we breathe is burnt with food and turned into energy. Our fireplace is the matrix. The place where ATP currency is obtained is the matrix.

In Plan B, however, energy is produced in the cytoplasm. While energy cannot be produced without oxygen in the mitochondria, it can be in the cytoplasm. In spite of that, the energy produced in the cytoplasm is both very little and harmful to the cell because of the waste it generates.

The amount of energy produced in the mitochondrial matrix is much more than that which is produced in the cytoplasm. Plan A energy is essential for a long life. Plan B is the method to obtain the energy used in emergencies. If we had been dependant on such a small amount of energy, this energy would not have enabled us to evolve over time and make us supreme human beings. **We would have remained as single cells.** Moreover, single-cell organisms still use this type of method for energy production.

The reason we have evolved is because we have been able to produce energy in the mitochondria with plan A!

Not content with the little energy obtained in the cytoplasm with Plan B, we have been evolving ever since we subsequently began to obtain more energy in the mitochondrial matrix. If we look after the mitochondria well and increase them, we will evolve even faster. As energy increases, we will be able to carry out more complex functions. **This book's purpose is to help us increase our speed in evolving.**

If the mitochondria do not perform well, not only

do we get ill but also our evolution slows down. If we are forced to settle with a small amount of energy in the cell cytoplasm because the mitochondrion is dysfunctional (like in single cells), we would regress in terms of our evolution. For instance, the cancer cell is a cell that has devolved in this way. It is a primitive cell that can use only sugar for energy and settles for the low energy in the cytoplasm, because it cannot produce energy in the mitochondria.

In a great many diseases, it is a question of damage in the performance of the mitochondria. **Health is proportionate to the capacity of the mitochondria's energy production. If we learn how a morsel of food is turned into energy in the cell through plans A and B, we will comprehend more clearly the matter of good health and disease.**

Energy is essential for the cell to stay alive—for it not to die. Normally, the extraction of energy from food starts first with Plan B, and then Plan A steps in. Let's take a closer look at them.

Plan B Survival Strategies

In Plan B, energy production does not occur in the mitochondria but in the cytoplasm. If the food is merely sugar, that is **glucose**, it can be converted into energy here whereas fat and proteins cannot.

Glucose first enters the cell with the help of *insulin* from the cell's outer membrane. Insulin combines with a structure in the cell membrane, called an *insulin receptor*, that belongs to it. The cell can only open its door to glucose in this way. Passing to the cell's cytoplasm, the glucose is converted into a product known as **pyruvate** through biochemical chain events. The process to obtain energy so far is Plan B. In Plan B, from glucose to pyruvate, a small amount of energy is produced. However, if this pyruvate is taken and sent to the mitochondrial matrix, the process moves on to Plan A and then a lot of energy can be produced. **It is this transition that creates the difference between health and disease.**

The energy model we always desire is energy production in the mitochondria, which we have identified as Plan A. For this to occur, the mitochondria have to be healthy and have enough oxygen. If this is not the case, pyruvate cannot pass to the mitochondria. If pyruvate cannot move to the mitochondria, it collects in the cell cytoplasm. To be able to produce energy there, with anaerobic respiration, it is converted into **lactate**. Therefore, pyruvate becomes lactate—in other words, **lactic acid**. Unfortunately, lactic acid is an end product we do not want.

If pyruvate in the cell cytoplasm can pass to the mitochondria, it goes through a biochemical process in the mitochondria called the **Krebs cycle**. The only thing we need to know about the Krebs cycle is the fact that it is the name for the transition of the energy production from Plan B to Plan A.

In brief:

- The medical term for Plan B energy production is glycolysis

- Plan B occurs in the cell's cytoplasm.

- In Plan B, oxygen is not needed—it is anaerobic.

- In Plan B, glucose is converted to pyruvate.

- In Plan B, two molecules of ATP are obtained from one molecule of glucose.

- If there is oxygen and the mitochondria are healthy, pyruvate moves to the mitochondria for Plan A energy production.

- The medical term for Plan A energy production is the Krebs cycle.

- In Plan A, thirty-four more molecules of ATP are obtained from pyruvate in the mitochondria.

- In Plan A, if our mitochondria are healthy, we obtain thirty-six ATP molecules from one glucose molecule.

- If the mitochondria are damaged or if there is no oxygen, it remains in Plan B; from one glucose molecule we obtain two ATP molecules.

- The result of Plan B is lactic acid.

- Plan B is the state of fermentation; in other words, obtaining energy through decomposition.

Note: While glucose can use both Plans A and B, fats never go through Plan B. Fat burn only occurs in the mitochondria; 129 ATP molecules are obtained from 1 molecule of fatty acid.

Let's now see how this high energy is obtained in the mitochondria.

Plan A Survival Strategies

In the Krebs cycle in mitochondria, the energy stored in food is decomposed, and this energy is finally collected in the hydrogen indicated with the letter H in a substance called **NADH (Nicotinamide adenine dinucleotide is the coenzyme's reduced state).** The final energy-form of the energy in food is this substance. (You may perhaps not be very familiar with these adjacent letters forming a chemical abbreviation. But, they were produced as the *vitamin supplement* by scientists interested in longevity and have since entered our lives.)

NADH is a carrier for electrons. Let me remind you that the energy in plants is stored as **electrons** in the atoms of leaves, seeds and fruits of plants. In other words, even though energy appears as food (such as an apple), energy is, in fact, kept in the electrons in the bonds between carbon atoms.

Whatever we eat, it is ultimately the electrons in food that turn into energy. It does not matter if it is bread, grapes, or yogurt; the final state is the same. Our complex digestive system and digestion, all our digestive organs such as the stomach and liver do, in fact, try to bring what is eaten into a state that can be transferred to NADH. None of us burns the apple in the mitochondria just because we ate the apple. We burn the electrons derived from the apple.

Set the Electrons on Fire

Using the electrons of food, the job of producing energy occurs in *the matrix, the mitochondrial membrane*. Here, oxygen steps in. The aim of breathing is to be able to produce energy with aerobic respiration. In order to obtain energy from electrons, they have to be oxidized. Oxidization begins with the high-energy electrons in food being burnt with air and being carried to lower energy electron-acceptors. **The difference in energy is used in the formation of ATP.** While energy is being obtained, carbon dioxide and water also result as the final product.

Food Electrons + Oxygen = Carbon Dioxide + Water +

ATP

At this stage, in order to obtain ATP, hydrogen molecules separate from the electron carriers carrying the food electrons inside them.

NADH = NAD + H

In other words, the H (hydrogen) in the NADH separates. This hydrogen is in any case the part carrying the energy of the food inside it.

NADH is the universal electron carrier. The food electrons in both plants and animals are carried by NADH. The job of obtaining energy in living things in the whole world occurs through the *hydrogen* of NADH. The proportion of NADH/NAD in mitochondria determines the energy capacity of mitochondria. Our aim in eating is to obtain the maximum NADH from food. The hydrogen of NADH carries the electrons that come from food. In all living creatures, energy is obtained through this hydrogen.

In order to obtain energy from hydrogen, hydrogen's atom is separated. Hydrogen is the simplest atom. It has a little proton p shown with a plus sign (+) and a little electron e shown with a minus sign (-).

The energy from the hydrogen's (-) negatively charged electron and the hydrogen's (+) positively charged proton is pumped outside the mitochondrial matrix membrane by a system called the **proton pump**. The name for this is the **electron transport chain (ETC).**

The ETC functioning properly is so determinative in aging and illness that it will become the most researched subject in medicine in the future.

While electrons are negatively (-) charged, protons are positively (+) charged. The positive (+) charge created by the protons pumped out of the matrix positively charges the outside of the membrane. *(So much detail may seem boring. But the secret to longevity is hidden in this matter of [+] and [-]).*

In conclusion, while one side of the matrix is full of protons, in other words positively charged (+), the other side of the membrane is not. This causes a difference in concentration. Because of this difference, protons want to quickly go from the place where they are in abundance towards the place where they are scarce. **Just as water that is pumped up and gushes down again like a waterfall with the pull of gravity in hydroelectric plants,** protons turn like a type of turbine as they pass from one side of the membrane to the other, similar to water turning the turbine in a plant and obtaining electricity with this movement. This turbine is the last stage where ATP is obtained.

Let's recall what we've learned so far…

Plants are exposed to the sun, and energy is collected in the plant's electrons.

↓

We eat plants and fruit, and food is digested.

↓

Food comes to the cell.

↓

In the cytoplasm, Plan B is completed.

↓

Mitochondria enters the scene and Plan A starts.

↓

The electrons in food are collected through NADH.

↓

Hydrogen is separated from NADH.

↓

The protons in the hydrogen are pushed outside of the matrix.

↓

The outside of the matrix becomes positively (+) charged and the inside negatively (-) charged.

↓

ATP is obtained through this difference.

RESULT: We eat the sun and obtain energy!

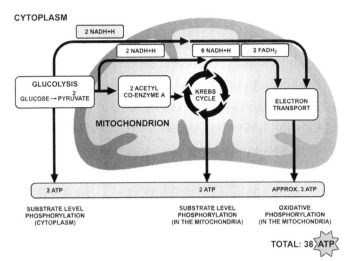

Figure 4: ATP production in the Mitochondria

So, we have finally reached the purpose of eating. We obtain energy.

Thank goodness.

However, food is not free. In nature, there is a price to pay…

Chapter 2:

TRADING IMMORTALITY FOR VITALITY

Free Radicals and Antioxidants

Since nutrition means that nutrients burn with oxygen, it would be shrewd to foresee the implication that, as with all combustion involving oxygen, a small amount of **ashes** will be produced. This is where the complexity of the matter begins. Ashes are harmful. They are waste. Rubbish. The biochemical name for these ashes is *free radicals*. Every single free radical is an anarchist.

The **antioxidants** and **free radicals**, which we have been reading about for years in every newspaper column, are related to energy production and diseases. In any case, whatever happens to us, it all comes from these free radicals.

Free radicals are the most important reason why we get ill and age!

Even if we seem to get ill or age for other reasons, that

is how the picture looks from the very top. The real view is on the atomic level, which shows that the fundamental common dominator between all sorts of diseases and aging is the damage inflicted by free radicals. The most important micro-prevention guaranteeing health and youth is ensuring that there is a minimum of free radicals.

Know Your Enemy Well: What Are Free Radicals?

What did I say earlier? That an atom contains electrons, protons, and neutrons. That the number of electrons and protons are equal. And that the protons are positively (+) charged and electrons are negatively (-) charged. This we know.

- If an atom has fewer electrons than protons, i.e., if there is a shortfall of electrons, the atom is positively (+) charged. This atom, which is lacking electrons, is called a *free radical.*

- If an atom has more electrons than protons, i.e., if it is negatively (-) charged, the atom is an *antioxidant*.

So, when the atom is positively (+) charged, it is a free radical. It is lacking electrons. The atom isn't balanced. An unbalanced atom is very aggressive. In a thousandth of a second, it will go and steal from the nearest electron provider. The source from which the electron is stolen will be damaged, but the free radical electron doesn't care. It is the antioxidant that gives the free radical the electron.

Free Radical = No Electron
Antioxidant = Many Electrons

This is a simple way to remember it.

In other words, when you hear statements such as "eat antioxidant foods" and about "this antioxidant and that antioxidant," it means that there are a lot of electrons in those nutrients, and we must realise that the **food can provide electrons**. These types of food are electron donors. The items you hear about in daily life that "create free radicals" (processed food, chemicals, preservatives, infections, polluted air, fried food, food cooked on a high heat like barbecues and cigarettes) signify that electrons will be stolen from the body.

Let's forget the free radicals that come from outside for the moment. Our subject now is what happens internally. Since energy production using oxygen mainly occurs in the cell's mitochondria, this is where most ashes will form. Indeed, the place that produces most free radicals in the body is in the mitochondria. Free radicals appear at the same time as ATP is produced. But, it is also in the mitochondria that the antioxidant defence mechanism is most efficient. Our body is a smart machine. However, the capacity of this antioxidant defence is limited.

The proportion of the antioxidants in mitochondria and free radicals determine both the quality and longevity of our lives. This matter of (+) and (-) is the secret to long life that we have been talking about. The (-) forming in the mitochondria are antioxidants and the (+) are free radicals. When the balance tips towards (+), in other words, when free radical production increases, diseases begin. **This is invariably the starting point in the micro-world of all diseases.**

Free Radicals Are the Price of Eating.

Eating is never a hundred percent beneficial; whatever you eat, there will always be some sort of damage. That is the law of nature. While we eat to live, unwanted "waste" formed at the end of the process will always accumulate over the years. Aging is an "accumulation of waste."

We come into the world by trading immortality for vitality. But the subject of our book is based on eating with **minimum damage and maximum benefit**.

- ✓ Maximum benefit means maximum work energy. This energy is to be used for repair, growth, and activity.
- ✓ Minimum damage means the waste, or the

rubbish, from the energy metabolism being kept at a minimum. This means minimum illnesses and maximum lifespan.

In short, if we have "an energy production system working with maximum benefit," our life will be optimal. **The obstacle to living forever is waste and lack of energy.**

Throughout this book, we will discuss how we can achieve this optimal living. But first, we have to understand why it is that there will always be some free radical damage no matter what we eat.

The Cost of Energy

We digest our food and send it on to the cell. In the cell, we obtain ATP first in the cytoplasm, then in the mitochondria—the cell's energy battery, and finally, in the mitochondrial membrane. It is this last part that is essential for vitality, because this is where the especially high energy is obtained, and this is where the price of energy is paid.

Let's remember that energy is simply that of the energy-charged electrons in foodstuffs. Let's remember that with this energy, the protons are **forcefully** pushed from one side of the membrane to the other. The positively (+) charged protons pumped out through the membrane make the outside of the membrane more positively (+) charged than inside of the membrane. Due to this difference in voltage, the protons are gushed inside like a waterfall from where there are many to where there are few—just like the turbine of a hydroelectric central. And this is how we obtain ATP.

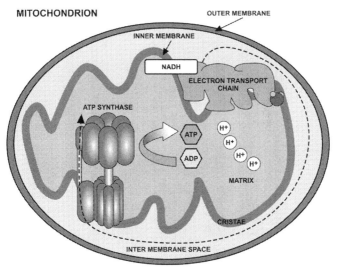

Figure 5: Energy Production in the Mitochondrion and Its Proton Pump

As it can be seen, the important point here is the ability of the positively charged (+) protons to be pushed outside the mitochondrial matrix membrane. Why are they pushed by force? The reason is that the mitochondrial membrane is not permeable for protons. They need to be pushed by energy. Now, let's stop here. What happens if these protons cannot be sufficiently pushed out of the membrane from the inside?

First of all, energy decreases because ATP

production decreases. It has not been possible to pump sufficient numbers of protons out of the matrix. It has not been possible to create the proton concentration difference outside the membrane. What else, apart from a decrease in energy, will happen if the positively (+) charged protons are not pushed out but remain inside? Will they just stay there like that, positively (+) charged? Won't they be looking for the negatively (-) charged electrons they are lacking? Aren't the positively charged atoms, those that are seeking the negative that they lack, what we call free radicals?

This is how the ashes (the free radicals), the price of burning nutrition with oxygen, materialize. While ATP is produced, there will always be a tiny leak of protons, i.e., a leak of free radicals. Under the most ideal conditions, even with the most ideal diet, the leak equals three in a thousand of the total energy. Normally, the attack of the free radicals also causes some damage.

- This happens with every breath.
- This is the cost of a life with oxygen.
- In our quest for energy, we are going to produce a little or a lot of free radicals.
- We have to cope with them.

Just as the heat energy from firewood produces smoke and ashes, we always produce some ash when we generate energy. **In any case, what we call aging is, in**

fact, an accumulation of ashes. What kind of nutrition makes good firewood and leaves little ash when burning, and which does not add too much to the natural and inevitable ashes we are bound to produce, is the subject we will deal with in this book.

Let's look at what happens to our health when these ashes accumulate in the hearth.

The free radicals are crazy, aggressive things. The name **radical** spells out that they have the power to destroy whatever comes their way. Since all they care about is finding the lacking electrons, they will attack the nearest and easiest target to obtain them.

The easiest place in the whole body where free radicals can obtain electrons is from the **lipid bilayer**, the membranes' **fatty acid. This knowledge is of vital importance.**

The most important organelles to be protected in the body are the cell membranes and the mitochondrial membranes. These are more important than both the heart and the brain!

You may think I'm exaggerating, but I am not. These organs are in any case formed by cells, too, and their cells are using the same energy metabolism. In fact, since they need more energy, they have a greater number of mitochondria than normal cells. Therefore, with regard to energy, these organs concede their goals to these free radicals, or terrorists.

Look Out! They Are Stealing Your Electrons!

The Voluntary Anti-Terror Unit It is the job of our cells

to protect the membranes from terrorists. Inherent in every cell are various ash cleaning systems protecting it against a free radical attack. These are our ***antioxidant*** systems. While the free radical causes damage by oxidizing (rusting), it is the antioxidant that stops it. It is the antioxidant that volunteers missing electrons to the free radical. When a free radical cannot find a volunteer donor, it will take a reluctant one regardless.

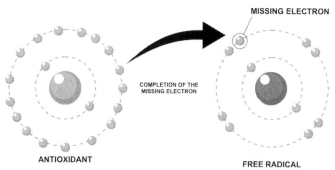

Figure 6: Antioxidants and Free Radicals

If there isn't a volunteer antioxidant, the cell membrane is the easiest place for the free radical to steal the electron. The mitochondrial membrane, that is the outer membrane surrounding the matrix and the mitochondria of the main cell, is an accessible target from which the electrons are stolen.

The stealing begins with electrons being stolen from the matrix. This is where the proton pumping takes place. If these protons are not pumped out, they will move as free radicals. They will attack the matrix—

the greatest terrorist formation hub.

Why do free radicals like the membranes? Let's take a quick look at that, too.

The Reluctant Anti-Terror Unit

All the cell membranes are rich in unsaturated fats. And that is how it should be. When the rate of unsaturated fat is high, the membrane is young. It is thin and pliable, and it is full of electrons. These electrons make the membrane thin and pliable. Whenever you hear the term "unsaturated fat," you should perceive it as **"proton unsaturation."** Unsaturated fat means that there are plenty of electrons. It means that protons (even if they are reluctant) can be saturated.

If the antioxidant systems within the cell are not sufficient, the cell membranes will be the first place from which the free radicals will steal electrons, as it is full of the electrons of the unsaturated fatty acids. The membranes serve as a kind of antioxidant, but reluctantly.

Death Comes with Rust

The free radicals take the fatty acids' electrons from inside the matrix and oxidize the membrane. They make it rusty. The membrane rusts. It becomes a bad membrane. Moreover, because energy production itself is also on the membrane, the energy production is also harmed. When there is free radical damage in the matrix, the ATP production slows down. That finishes off the energy. As a result, the cell that cannot produce energy in the mitochondria dies. **This is because the formation of free radicals and the membrane damage continues in a vicious cycle.**

If the membrane is damaged by free radicals, the following occurs:

- The electrons on the membrane decrease, the membrane becomes thick and hard. The membrane rusts.

- The uptake of oxygen in the mitochondria slows down because all of the oxygenated ATP energy is obtained through the membrane.

- The speed of the proton pump that pumps the protons out of the membrane slows down.

- Protons, i.e., free radicals, accumulate on the membrane.

- The membrane rusts even more.

- The formation of ATP slows down and finally stops.

- The mitochondrion decides to die

- New mitochondria are made to replace it.

The name of this cell death is **apoptosis**. This means **"planned cell-suicide,"** and this is very valuable to us; it is something that preserves our health. Which of our organs would want badly functioning mitochondria? It is a good thing that the bad mitochondria are removed, as new ones must take their place. It is the mitochondria that decide the suicide of damaged cells. Mitochondria are social. If the mitochondria are damaged, they sacrifice themselves for the common good. In cases where the planned cell-suicide (apoptosis) is impaired, it causes illnesses and cancer. **Cancer cells are egoistic. Rather than thinking about the common good, they try to grow by destroying the whole.** Apoptosis is the only way for us to regenerate and not be content with the old.

However, the renewal of mitochondria becomes harder as we get older. And when the mitochondria cannot be renewed, we have to put up with cells that function badly or tolerate less energy than we used to have. **This means that we must care better for our mitochondria as we age!** We should protect them much more from free radical damage. Damage to the mitochondria means an increased leak of free radicals.

Therefore, both the body's own antioxidants and the antioxidants obtained from our foodstuffs become indispensable. If there are not enough antioxidants, the price will be paid by damage to the membranes. If the cells with bad membranes die through apoptosis, it is fine. Later new copies of these bad cells will replace them. But as this copying becomes more frequent, in time there will be **"bad copies of a bad copy."**

If a bad copy of a cell is made or if a new copy of a cell that has committed suicide cannot be made, it probably means we have become old. When we are young, there are many mitochondria and much more energy for the same tasks. But as we get older, we will not have enough of either energy or mitochondria. The mitochondria of a 90-year-old person have decreased by 50% compared to those of a 20-year-old. Few mitochondria mean little energy. Little energy means little activity and little repair.

Batteries Deplete As We Grow Old

Diseases do not, of course, develop in a day. The damage that we have been describing accumulates in the cell over the years, and eventually diseases develop in the organs. **Therefore, serious illnesses emerge with aging with the accumulation of badly functioning cells. This is why cancer, for example, occurs more frequently as we grow older.**

The cancer cell is, in fact, nothing more than a smart cell trying to survive under difficult conditions. In order not to die, they push the limits so hard that instead of producing energy like sophisticated human cells, they do it through fermentation or decomposition like unicellular organisms. Once again, it is (for whatever reason) primarily the increasing free radical damage.

If the mitochondrial membrane is damaged by the leak of free radicals, it cannot obtain any electrons from the ETC. If the ETC does not work, it won't be possible to produce energy in the aerobic Plan A. Then, all we have is Plan B energy production. This means lactic acid will emerge from the pyruvate produced from glycose. Lactic acid, as its name indicates, is an acid. **As it accumulates, the pH of the cell that should be alkali turns acidic. Acidic pH reduces the oxygen used for the cell's energy.** The cell that tries to survive opts to use much more glucose, which is the only matter from which the cell can obtain energy without oxygen. As it continues to obtain energy in the cytoplasm from glycose, the acid will increase and the accumulating damage will also affect the cell's DNA. Eventually, the cell will begin to reproduce out of control. **This is what we call cancer. Cancer is simply mitochondrial damage. And yet, the cell hasn't committed the planned cell-suicide, apoptosis.** When the damaged cell's apoptosis mechanisms don't work and the cell doesn't die, it will reproduce uncontrollably.

What Are Our Trump Cards That Will Save Us from Disaster?

In light of all this information, we should ask the following pertinent question: what can we do to keep our mitochondria and membranes healthy? First of all, we must make the right choice of food. **We can choose nutrition that contains many electrons, meaning plenty of antioxidants. We can replace the fatty acids of the membranes.** Then we can change our lifestyles: optimize our sleep, do exercise, and give up smoking. These are our weapons. These are the cards we have up our sleeves in order to control our **"fates."**

If we know our biology well—or as we have learned from the explanations what we now call **quantum biology**—and abide by the rules, we can embrace a very long life.

Why Is the Name of This Book "Quantum Nutrition"?

Very simple. When it's a question of interaction between subatomic particles such as electrons and protons in biology, the rules are determined by quantum biology, not classical biology.

- *Electrons are tiny, little quantum things.*
- *The purpose of eating is to obtain electrons (-)*
- *Protons are also tiny, little quantum things.*
- *The reason for illnesses is proton (+) damage.*
- *Life is nothing more than plus (+) and minus (-) charges.*

However, balance is not what is desired here. Minuses must always outnumber pluses. Minuses are needed for energy. When these two are in balance or when pluses outnumber minuses, it means death.

Life Is the Current of Bioelectricity

When the plus (+) charges on both sides of the

mitochondrial membrane are equal—when there is balance—the flow of protons stops. This is because the electrical charges are equal and then there is no slope. In other words, there is no difference in the electrical charges. Then, there can be no ATP production either. When the electric current stops, we are dead. All creatures whose electric current has stopped die. Death is the ceasing of the bioelectrical flow.

This means that for a good electric current, we need:

- ✓ Electrons in the food

- ✓ Oxygen

- ✓ Good membranes

We can only obtain the necessary ATP by producing electrical energy. **The purpose of this book is to help you increase the electrons that protect your electricity. Food is, in fact, acquiring fuel for the bioelectrical current.**

Do we have the luxury then to say, "I don't want to become stressed out about food. So what if my electricity flows slowly?"

Chapter 3:

THE SINGLE COMMON MECHANISM OF ALL DISEASES

Every Disease Begins for the Same Reason: The Deterioration of the Mitochondria

Do you worry about your spots? Have you recovered from cancer? Or, do your age spots or hyperthyroid make you unhappy? **Although they seem incomparable, every disease begins more or less for the same reason: deterioration of the mitochondria.**

If the cells haven't broken down, then why should the organ get ill? Well, why do cells break down? Even if we gather a great many factors under different headings, we always arrive at the same point.

- the wrong foods for energy production in the cell (bad fuel for the engine)

- free radicals that occur while energy is being produced (too many exhaust fumes)

- the inability to sufficiently clean up free radicals (a blocked exhaust)

- cell membranes damaged by free radicals (exhaust damaging the engine)

- decrease in energy for work and repair (the car not going because the energy from the engine has decreased)

As the result of all of the above, diseases and aging occur as the years progress. If we are to consider it more simply, the whole process boils down to the increase in waste production and decrease in waste excretion.

Wherever you find the bad chain listed above, that organ is already ill. By the time you notice the disease, it would have begun to develop along with the faults in this chain. And the build-up of damaged cells increases so much that now one of your organs is diseased.

I wondered how many names of diseases there are in the world. I was curious about this; according to Google, it is thirty thousand. The names of the diseases may be different: diabetes, hyperthyroidism, polycystic ovaries, cancer, and so on, but the basic beginning is the same. Everything begins in one single cell. Anything to the contrary can happen only in the case of accidents, not diseases. In that case, we must know what that single cell is like when healthy so that we can prevent it from breaking down.

What Is a Healthy Cell like?

Let's keep in mind that we have forty trillion cells. Some characteristics of cells must be complete in order for us to be able to identify them as healthy cells.

First Rule for a Healthy Cell: The Membranes Must Be Healthy!

The membranes of the cells must be thin and pliable!

This pliancy and thinness depends on the amount of omega-3 fatty acids in the membrane. If the omega-3 fatty acids are more than omega-6, then the membrane is thin and pliable. There are plenty of electrons in omega-3 fatty acids. An abundance of electrons is desired in all membranes. The presence of electrons protects the membrane against oxidation. They prevent the cell from hardening. If the amount of omega-3 decreases in the cells, the membranes begin to harden. The hardening of the membrane is what all diseases have in common.

The doors of the outer membrane of the cell must be strong!

The cell membrane keeps the inside and the outside (of the cell) at a different ion concentration. The electric charge inside the cell differs from that on the outside of the cell. This difference creates an electric voltage on the cell membrane. In other words, the top of the cell membranes are electrical. The difference in inner and outer voltage normally keeps the doors closed. If the cell wants something to enter, it changes the voltage and opens the door and then closes it. These electrical valves open and close with biochemical methods called the sodium potassium pump and ion channels.

If I say that twenty-five percent, a quarter of this energy, which we obtain from the food we eat and drink every day and whose importance I've so far greatly emphasized, is spent on opening and shutting these doors, I think you will understand the importance of the locks. So much energy is consumed here, because inserting stuff into a cell and disposing the rubbish from inside is a very important job that requires energy. What we need to know is that it is imperative for the membrane-doors to work well, and that this will be ensured by a healthy membrane.

The hormone locks on the outer membrane of the cell must be strong!

On the cell membranes, there are hormone receptors that act in a similar way to locks. By recognizing the hormones that appear and by responding to them appropriately, these receptors work like a type of lock. For the hormones to give a command to the cells, they have to fit the lock exactly, just as a key would. Hormones in a healthy cell membrane alert the Lego-like receptors and fit perfectly like lock and key.

Without the lock and key alignment, the hormone cannot give the cell work to do. Besides, when the cell membranes harden and lose their pliancy and thinness, these receptors (or locks) will not be compatible with their own keys. The simplest example is the condition called **insulin resistance**, which we hear about repeatedly. The lock fitting the insulin hormone has broken. We will return to this subject in more detail later.

As with the cell membrane, mitochondrial membranes must also be thin!

The electron transport chain (ETC) in the matrix is of vital importance. If we have been able to bring the electrons in food this far, the sturdiness of this membrane is essential for us to burn it with oxygen and produce ATP. Remember that protons are pumped from inside this membrane to the outside, after which ATP is formed. This membrane has to be thin for the protons to be easily pumped outside the membrane; otherwise, protons collecting inside will cause free radical damage, and this damage will eventually kill the cell.

The Second Rule for a Healthy Cell: Antioxidant Mechanisms Must Work Well!

The main reason for damage is an increase in free radicals and an inadequate antioxidant system. There are some antioxidant systems in the cell, of which we know the names—**glutathione, selenium, superoxide**

dismutase, and these are busy 24/7. The aforementioned NADH also functions as an antioxidant as it carries the electrons that come with the food, and electrons are antioxidants.

However, glutathione is the most important of these antioxidants. In any event, the others assist glutathione. Glutathione is our most important raw material cleaning out the free radicals in the cell and mitochondrion. Suggestions for nutrition to increase glutathione and other antioxidants will be given later in the book. These antioxidants must always be able to do sufficient free-radical cleaning. The refuse collectors must work well.

The Third Rule for a Healthy Cell: The Cell Must Be Able to Repair Itself!

As well as having good membranes and a good waste-cleaner, the healthy cell must have the capacity to be able to repair itself.

The Fourth Rule for a Healthy Cell: It Must, If Necessary, Be Able to Sacrifice Itself for the Greater Good!

This is exactly where *apoptosis* and *autophagy* step in. You may recall that apoptosis can be defined as the cell's self-destruction in the event that the damage to the cell cannot be repaired. *Autophagy*, however, is the destruction of unhealthy cells by being cannibalized by the other cells of the body.

Both these methods are significant ways to dispose

of aged or diseased cells. And both these systems have to work extremely well. In failing to do so, incompetent cells with accumulated waste that produce little energy will reduce the functions of the organs. The name of this state is disease.

Let's recall in simple terms what has been explained in this part:

- Diseases begin from the mitochondria.

- The free radicals in the mitochondria not being cleaned is the reason for disease.

- The free radicals' first target of attack is the membranes.

- Membranes give electrons to free radicals as an antioxidant.

- A membrane that loses its electrons rusts.

- Damage to the membrane is one of the common starting points of all diseases.

- In nutrition, the right fuel must be chosen for the mitochondria.

- If it has plenty of electrons, that food is an antioxidant.

- If it has few electrons, that food is a free radical.

In conclusion, if we have enough electrons, we could

perhaps be immortal. At this moment our greatest strength on the path to a long and healthy life is the power to be able to make our food choices for energy production for the good of our mitochondria.

The form of nutrition for the good of our mitochondria, known by its popular name as alkaline diet or alkaline nutrition, is given top attention in this book—which focuses on quantum alkaline nutrition.

What Is pH?

We are made to remember our pH balance again. The essence of the matter is in comprehending this part. pH is the amount of the hydrogen proton (+) charge. It may seem complicated, but it is actually extremely simple: **wherever there are a lot of hydrogen protons (+), that place is acidic. Contrarily, wherever there are a lot of hydrogen electrons (-), that place is alkaline. After all, we have been talking about hydrogen protons and electrons since the beginning of the book. Now let's combine this information.**

The pH value is shown on a scale of 0 to 14. A value of acidity is pH 7 and below. If the number of positively (+) charged protons in a fluid or tissue are more, that fluid or tissue is acidic. Let's never forget that protons mean free radicals.

- acidification

- increase in protons

- increase in positive (+) charges

- increase in free radicals

These are all the same.

Alkalinity, the opposite of acidity, is as follows: if there are few positive (+) charges in a fluid or tissue, and consequently, there are more negative (-) charges in the environment, then the pH is above 7. In other words, there are more electrons. When there are more electrons, we know to identify them as antioxidants.

- to be alkaline

- increase in electrons

- increase in negative (-) charges

- increase in antioxidants

These too are all the same. In that case, in brief, **acidification** means the increase of free radicals, and **alkalinity** means a surplus of antioxidants.

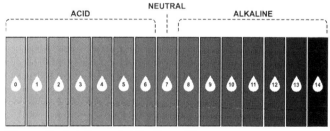

Figure 7: Acidic and Alkaline pH

When we refer to alkaline foods, we are referring to

antioxidant foods, which increase the number of electrons in the body. Now, it is not at all difficult to understand what is good food, is it? **In short, if it provides us with many electrons, then it's good food. Full stop.**

When our body is healthy, it is alkaline. The fluids inside, outside, and between the cells are at the alkaline pH level.

The place that I must particularly stress here again is the mitochondrial matrix membrane. This is because the most alkaline fluid in the body is in the matrix. Normally, the matrix is the place where the fewest positive (+) charges are kept due to the protons being pumped outside. The pH here is between 8 and 8.5. The body's most alkaline cell structure is here, and only if it stays like this can we produce enough energy.

The whole aim of this book is to show the way to preserve the matrix's alkaline pH with diet and life style suggestions. Here lies the secret of longevity.

Certain support systems are switched on to protect the matrix's alkaline pH in all the cells. **The acid buffer systems** constantly work with all their might in order to keep the whole body at an alkaline pH. In order to maintain the desired pH, these buffer systems try to reduce the proton charge, i.e., the free radical charges.

To summarize, there must be few free radicals in the body. This is simple and logical. If there are more positive (+) charges, they will take the negative (-) ones they need from the membranes and damage the membranes. In such a case, first the mitochondrial membranes, where the positive (+) charge was first formed, will no longer be able to function. If the mitochondria do not work well, the Plan A high energy production, where oxygen is used, will cease to work. We will not be able to use the fatty acids and proteins for energy, either. If the mitochondria do not work, we will be dependent on Plan B, which produces little energy in the cytoplasm. Here, only **sugar** is utilized, and the energy obtained is not enough. With the increase in the amount of lactic acid, the consequence is more acidification.

If energy cannot be produced in the mitochondria, and we are forced into energy production in the cytoplasm, the lactic acid formed will acidify the intracellular pH. **Acidification and free radical increase are the same.** Free radicals beginning in the mitochondria and advancing to the cytoplasm will now attack the outer membrane of the cell. Because there are unsaturated omega-3 fatty acids with plenty of electrons in the outer membrane, the free radicals will begin to steal electrons from there. **The reason behind the insufficient functioning of the mitochondria is oxidation of the cell's outer membrane.** Ultimately, the cell's outer membrane, which needs to be thin and pliable—in other words the cell's main entrance door, also hardens.

All diseases progress with the hardening of

the cell's outer membrane.

This is because the food—in other words, the raw materials providing the energy—enter the cell through this membrane, and the rubbish exits the same place. All hormones give commands through the receptors on top of the cell's outer membrane. As the membrane breaks down, so does the chain of command.

As free radicals (acidification) continue to increase, there is damage to the cell's nucleus.

↓

Our DNA (where our vital data is kept) is in the nucleus.

↓

The increase of free radical damage and acidification can eventually also damage DNA.

↓

This can cause the cell to alter and become cancerous.

The name of the disease is not important. What is important is that they all begin in this way. As the condition progresses, a diagnosis is given according to the organ where there is damage.

Now shall we take a look at some of the most heard of diseases?

Chapter 4:

HOW DOES EACH DISEASE DEVELOP?

Aging

Even the healthiest looking among us cannot escape the aging that happens over the years. In general, we may not have a complaint. Nevertheless, our skin wrinkles, our hair turns gray, our mobility slows down, and our memory slows down. If we were to take a closer look at our aging organs by zooming in with a microscope, this is what we would see:

- Metabolic waste in our cells that hasn't been eliminated; for example, wrinkled hands and brain plaques found in patients with Alzheimer's.

- The mitochondria count in all our cells has decreased. We must now perform the same tasks but with fewer mitochondria. This means that our energy for work and repair has diminished. We now have mitochondria that move more slowly, tire more easily, and get less work done.

- The increase in free radical leakage in our mitochondria—the interesting discovery about aging.

Aging means that all activities and repair mechanisms appear to function in slow-motion. This is because the energy that normally provides pace has dwindled. Even by eating very well, we may not regain that energy. When our mitochondria diminish or cannot perform their functions very well, we cannot be as energetic as we would like. **In fact, we gain weight from most of what we eat because we cannot burn it.**

We should not measure our age in years but by the free radical leakage in our mitochondria. Mice, for instance, have substantial free radical leakage in their mitochondria. This is why their lifespan is limited to one or two years. Towards the end of their lives, they succumb to diseases associated with aging. In birds, however, there is only a small amount of free radical leakage; therefore, they live much longer and do not display any age-related diseases. **The lifespan of living creatures corresponds to their level of energy production and their free radical leakage.**

A treatment aimed at preventing the leaking of

free radicals may be, without exception, the single treatment for all age-related diseases.

The *mitochondrial theory of aging* and *free radical theory of aging are two most popular theories.* According to these theories, the mitochondria are our biological clocks, and leakage of electrons from the electron transport chain (ETC) is at the heart of aging. I agree with these ideas.

If the foods—the bad fuel we have consumed over the years—have caused a lot of damage, we must change our diet at once. We must immediately turn to an energy model that produces less exhaust. **If we replace cheap fuel such as sugar with alkaline foodstuffs, we can renew our decrepit cells.** Food that makes the body alkaline means food that contains electrons, i.e., antioxidants. This is food with minimal waste—unprocessed food. Using purer and additive-free fuel will increase our energy. Our biological clocks will begin to turn back time. When there are so many medical opportunities and much scientific knowledge, we should stop regretting the chronological advance of our years and concentrate on our biological age. This is done through alkaline nutrition and by adopting an alkaline lifestyle.

Anti-aging is a question of engine and fuel: staying young depends simply on that! The principle of alkaline eating is frequently repeated in this book, as well in my other two books. It's easy to learn and implement.

Non-dietary cell rejuvenation (specific vitamin supplements and intravenous cocktails) is supervised by a doctor. In all approaches, the aim is to decrease the cell's proton charge and increase its electron-antioxidant capacity. This is because aging and all existing diseases begin at this level.

Insulin Resistance

Insulin resistance and hyperglycemia, or type 2 diabetes, are related. I will discuss all of them individually.

You may hear a lot of people identify themselves as insulin resistant. This is because it has become commonplace. Formerly, it was overweight people over the age of forty-five who were diagnosed with insulin resistance. Nowadays, it is seen in children and people with a normal weight as well. Yet, patients do not understand exactly what this diagnosis entails.

There are similarities between insulin resistance, hypoglycaemia, and type 2 diabetes. They are merely the same disease at different stages. The underlying cause is the same and very simple.

Insulin is a hormone that wants to convey its commands to the cells, which it does through a special **insulin receptor** in the outer membrane of the cell. The insulin receptor adjusts to the insulin hormone like a key in a lock. **If there are more free radicals than the antioxidant-systems can capture, they will damage the cell membranes where the receptors are located;**

the free radicals oxidize the cell membranes. (A reminder: our cell membranes are covered in plenty of unsaturated fatty acids. It would be more correct to remember the fatty acids as "proton unsaturated." They may reluctantly surrender to the free radicals the missing electron that they are pursuing.)

When the free radicals steal electrons from the cell membranes, they cause a damaging chain reaction. Losing their electrons, the cell membranes lose their pliancy and become more rigid. The fit between the old insulin locks on the cell membranes—less pliable and more rigid than before—and insulin becomes more difficult. The insulin key can no longer find the lock as easily in order to introduce energy into the cell. **Even if it finds it, it won't be able to unlock the rusty lock.**

This simple explanation is very close to reality. When the lock does not open as readily as it used to, the blood sugar level in the pancreas falls to normal value with greater difficulty than before and, quite understandably, thinks we have **eaten more**. If we have insulin resistance, our pancreas thinks we are eating a lot. It does not care about the rusty lock that doesn't open. All it cares about is to quickly purify the blood, which is sticky like sugared water, and make it clear again. Because the pancreas doesn't know of the time wasted due to the unyielding rusty lock, it thinks that we are eating more than normal. As a result, it releases more insulin as it monitors the blood sugar level.

In addition, if the individual suffers from leaky gut

syndrome, or if they eat very quickly, the amount of sugar mixing with the blood will always look greater in a period of time. In such a situation, the amount of sugar mixing with the blood will be higher compared to someone who eats more slowly or whose gut is healthy. Furthermore, when simple carbohydrates are added to such a scenario, it makes matters worse. **Since simple floury and sugary foods are easily digested, they enter the bloodstream very swiftly.**

For all these reasons, when the insulin in the blood is high, insulin resistance will be diagnosed. However, the most important point here is that neither the pancreas nor the insulin is to be blamed. It isn't quite right to qualify the insulin as inactive, either. **The correct conclusion is that it slows down the impact-mechanism in the cells of the organ that the insulin is targeting.** If insulin, as a hormone, does not join the receptor, it struggles to do its job. And the receptor isn't the culprit here, either.

The real villains are the free radicals that oxidize, or rust, the membranes!

So, when you are told that "you have insulin resistance," you need to understand that free radicals have damaged your cell membranes, and that in order to minimize the free radicals, you need antioxidants— in other words, alkaline nutriments.

Hypoglycemia

Hypoglycemia is similarly the progression of the

mechanism mentioned in the section above. This is the situation before **full-blown diabetes**, which is created by the increased amount of insulin pushing at the rigid door in front of the cell membrane.

Once insulin leaves the pancreas, it does not return even after having completed its task. It will continue to perform its duties until the level reaches fasting insulin level. Since its first task is to lower the blood glycose level, it will do whatever it takes to accomplish the job. Moreover, since the amount of insulin in the amount of food we used to eat to feed our cells no longer suffices, due to the hardened membranes, we now have to cope with more insulin. Yet, you continue to eat just as before. **So, will the surplus insulin stop as it used to once the blood sugar reaches the normal fasting level? The answer is "no"— insulin is persistent**. It will work overtime and lower the blood glucose level to below normal fasting level. From the second hour after a meal, mostly in the third hour, you may experience some or all of these symptoms of hypoglycemia:

- drowsiness
- sugar cravings
- mental confusion
- chills
- trembling hands

When you go to the doctor with the above symptoms,

he or she will usually advise you to **eat more frequently. This, however, escalates the vicious cycle.** Whenever you eat, you will start the insulin-hypoglycemia chain.

In many cases, patients with hypoglycemia feel better when they don't eat; as a result, they feel more clear-headed and don't experience the hypoglycaemia symptoms. In other words, the hypoglycemia they don't have when fasting, emerges when they eat. **The significance of this is that our cell membranes cannot let our insulin-based food enter in order to turn it into energy. The cell within is hungry, but it stores the food as fat.** Even if we eat only a little bit of this type of food, we will put on weight.

Let's stop here and remind ourselves what the cells like to use as fuel for energy. We have trillions of mitochondria, which mean a high level of energy. We know that the source from which mitochondria receive energy is the electrons in the food. Foods with the most electrons are vegetables.

Once again, it is up to us to apply simple logic: since the outer membranes are damaged and won't pay attention to the insulin, we must eat food that does not need insulin.

However rigid the membranes, vegetables avoid the membranes as they enter the cell.

↓

Vegetables go directly to the mitochondria and are used for good energy production.

↓

Vegetables have plenty of electrons and fill the environment with antioxidants.

↓

These antioxidants stop the free radicals that cause the hardening of the membranes.

↓

Antioxidants replace the stolen electrons of the cell.

↓

Wherever there are plenty of electrons, pH will be alkaline (as is desired).

↓

The mitochondrial matrix that has now become alkaline produces plenty of ATP.

↓

You feel energetic and happy.

We can implement all this with regard to nearly every disease. Even knowing this much will help us throughout life in understanding the reasons for many disorders. Otherwise, the story will not end here. If you do not overcome insulin resistance or hypoglycemia, it will progress into diabetes.

Type 2 Diabetes

Type 2 diabetes develops after the two prior diagnoses, and it has become widespread throughout the whole world, even among the young. First there is insulin resistance, then hypoglycaemia, and finally type 2 diabetes. These are, in fact, all the same thing. It is just a question of increased damage, and this damage is in the cell membrane.

If you have been diagnosed with type 2 diabetes, it means that despite the efforts of the pancreas and all the insulin it has secreted, the cell membranes have become so hardened that the blood sugar cannot be brought back down to normal. The test for fasting insulin level shows approximately the amount of insulin waiting at the door of the cell. The amount of insulin waiting at the door as a key shows how rusted the locks have become.

The amount of fasting insulin gives away the aging of the cell!

However, merely avoiding carbohydrates is not the solution to rejuvenate our cells. Carbohydrates and simple sugars are generally the first restrictions given in the case of diabetes or in efforts to lose weight. This is an entirely correct approach. Indeed, no one, including our children, needs to eat these foodstuffs. **But we cannot make our hardened cell membranes more pliable by simply cutting out carbohydrates and sugars.** We have to look at the bigger picture and once more recognize the actual starting point.

The whole matter began with free radicals stealing electrons from the membranes. Since that is the case, we must restrict all nutritional sources that increase the production of free radicals that steal the electrons. All processed foods as well as carbohydrates and sugar belong to this group. Examples include processed meats, such as salami and ham, and even fried broccoli. **Even broccoli, if we fry it, becomes exactly like other bad foods that produce free radicals.** There seems to be no end to counting bad foodstuffs. The simplest thing to do is to focus on the good ones.

Thus, if we are talking about diabetes, insulin metabolism, or hypoglycaemia, the solution is always the same: vegetables full of electrons, unprocessed healthy animal products, and good oils.

The body is in fact such a comprehensive system that if one part is broken, it damages the whole. You may be insulin resistant simply because you cannot breathe properly through your nose at night. By solving somebody's sleep apnea problem, thereby allowing them to uptake sufficient oxygen, both their cholesterol levels and their insulin resistance will fall. That is not such earth-shattering information though. At this point in the book, you should be able to sense the flow:

If there is apnea, there is little oxygen.

If there is little oxygen, the energy production in the

mitochondria is low.

If the mitochondria do not work well, there are too many free radicals.

Electrons are stolen from the membranes.

Disease sets in.

This chain always follows the same logic.

Alzheimer's

Alzheimer's is now known in medical literature as **type 3 diabetes.** It is caused by years of irregular glycose peaks—in other words, sudden raised sugar levels that wear out the brain. **Alzheimer's can be said to be a long-term "sugaring" of the brain.** The term sugaring already exists in medicine and is also known as caramelization, which is a type of accumulation of free radical waste—also known with its medical name, **advanced glycation endproducts (AGEs).** The AGEs forming in the brain are caused by Alzheimer's special plaques. Biochemically, there is not a big difference between them and age spots, or liver spots on the skin. The areas in the brain with plaques cannot function properly, as the mitochondria in the areas with plaques are damaged.

Central to diseases that change brain functions,

such as Parkinson's, attention deficit disorder, dementia, brain fog, depression, reduced hearing, autism, and Alzheimer's, there is a problem with the brain's energy production and its damage-repair mechanism. The brain uses twenty percent of the body's energy. Because of this great need for energy, the brain cells contain far more mitochondria than other cells in the body. However, when their mitochondria are damaged, the energy in the brain diminishes. Without mitochondria the brain can utilize neither sugar nor fat. **All neurological diseases are accompanied by mitochondrial damage.**

In relevant literature, we can read that in the nutrient support and treatment of Alzheimer's at the moment, animal food products have been restricted; carbohydrates, sugar and processed foods have been removed; and vegetable foods and especially good vegetable oils have been added. This knowledge should be applied to all neurological and brain diseases.

In any case, when was cake, pie, cookies, spaghetti, pizza, rice, dessert, salami, ham, alcohol, and the like, ever recommended as treatment for an illness? Applying this simple logic isn't difficult for any of us. The whole purpose of this book is to persuade you to replace the above mentioned **"foods"** that cause acidification—in other words, those that create free radicals—with alkaline foods.

Polycystic Ovary Syndrome

Polycystic ovary syndrome is increasing with unprecedented speed. Seen in all women—young and mature—the symptoms are irregular periods, excess body hair, acne, hair loss, and ovarian cysts. Let's encapsulate the symptoms below:

- Despite being a woman, she experiences hair loss.

- Despite being a woman, she experiences excess body hair.

- Periods become irregular or cease altogether.

- Despite being past puberty, she has acne .

Here, I've used the word "woman" deliberately. For wouldn't you agree that the symptoms mentioned above do not indicate the female hormone estrogen but rather the male hormone testosterone?

Polycystic ovary syndrome is, in fact, not different from insulin resistance; **the former usually occurs alongside the latter.** Nevertheless, it is still a question of the membrane's rigidity and of an inactive hormone. As with insulin resistance, when the key no longer fits the lock, the hormones cannot give their commands to the inside of the cells.

The same case stands with estrogen, as it struggles to give commands through the hardened membranes. As the effect of estrogen decreases, the effect of testosterone appears to be greater.

With polycystic ovary syndrome, the commands

of estrogen don't reach their target. Both testosterone values as well as insulin values may be high in these individuals. For treatment, prescription of the contraceptive pill is recommended to boost the effect of estrogen. That is the subject of endocrinologists and gynecologists, however. What I want to explain here is that with regards to polycystic ovary syndrome, there is a problem with the hormone receptor, for which the solution is the same as that of insulin resistance. Apart from medical treatment, an alkaline diet model based on vegetables and vegetable fats, in order to protect the membranes, would assist in recovery—as with all other cases of hormone receptor disorders.

Do not forget:

- If your sleep is poor, your sleep is related to the hormone melatonin.

- If you are a man with a low libido, libido is related to the hormone testosterone

- If you are unhappy, happiness is related to the hormone serotonin

- Having mentioned "the happiness hormone," let's now take a look at the diseases affecting the area where it is produced.

Irritable Bowel Syndrome

If our subject is nutrition, the first place in the body where they are processed—the digestive system—

deserves special interest. **There is no rule saying that bad foods only create problems once they enter the cells. In actuality, they create problems for us from the very first bite.** Gastrointestinal disorders are probably the most widespread problems today. People with complaints such as constipation, indigestion, flatulence, and bloating used to go from one doctor to another; but nowadays, they can learn, at least to some degree, which foods to avoid.

In fact, we always somehow reach the right conclusion that in all illnesses it is the same foods we should avoid. When we consume these kinds of foods, they first damage the place where they enter the body. As a place of devastation, the intestines are already a very important area; and when this area is damaged, the effect on the body becomes quite significant.

With an absorption surface of up to four-hundred square meters, the immune system in the gut decides whether the food is detrimental to the body or not. The surface of the intestines, like the cell membranes, is selectively permeable. It tries to allow only that which it finds suitable to pass. To carry out this task, it is densely covered with small elongated projections called **"villi."**

These small projections try to prevent the absorption of unwanted foods. To achieve this, they are stuck together, allowing no space between them. However, if the corrugated and continuous surface begins to perforate, they may leak unwanted food. **Many allergic reactions are caused by degeneration**

of the impermeability in the intestines.

The impermeability of the intestines can be destroyed, as food that increases acidity causes local inflammation in the gut. **We can refer to the inflammation as a kind of "agonizing death" in that area. It desires to heal but cannot; it cannot manage to recover.** If you do not remove the agents (the foods) that are causing the disturbance, healing cannot take place. **The biochemical elements of the inflammation are free radicals, also known as protons.**

The reason why long drawn-out inflammation causes future diseases is excessive free radical damage in that area. Diseases such as leaky gut, ulcerous colitis, Crohn's disease, and so on, are local inflammatory diseases of the gut. Even one day of constipation can increase the number of free radicals that lead to inflammation of the gut. The increased number of free radicals will damage the cells' mitochondria and thus diminish energy production. The absorption of food, constriction of the gut to evacuate, and renewal of all the cells in the gut every three days are activities that need energy.

Local inflammation in the gut, or rather an attempt to repair damage that somehow does not succeed, will spread to other parts of the body if it isn't prevented from doing so. If there are other parts in the body that haven't been repaired, the attempts at healing will proceed from bad to worse. This situation exacerbates

autoimmune illnesses since inflammation sustains autoimmune diseases.

It is the emergence of the inflammatory matters that make the inflammation as bad as it is; they propagate the free radicals in the environment. Thyroid disorders can be given as an example of inflammations far removed from the gut. This disease can be caused by inflammation or by the proteins in the thyroid gland attacking the body.

The mitochondria in the inflamed cells become damaged, leading to the fall of energy production. But, energy is necessary for repair.

Inflammation should be prevented at the point of digestion. Let's see how some simple suggestions can help the gastrointestinal tract.

1. *First of all, you have to increase chewing! Don't forget, you haven't got teeth in your stomach!*

We do not pay enough attention to chewing. Our mouth and teeth are for breaking down the food before it can be fed to a tiny organ at micro level, such as the mitochondria. The more you chew, the better the food is broken down and the fewer the enzymes needed for digestion. This protects our pancreas.

Because of the effort put into chewing more meticulously, the time it takes for energy to enter the bloodstream will be extended. Since the food will enter the gut more slowly, we can control weight gain—even if we eat unhealthy foods. You may notice that all reluctant eaters are slim. If you chew properly, you will have fewer flatulence and constipation complaints.

2. You should avoid eating acidifying foods!

We know that fast food, fried food, alcohol, flour- and sugar-based foods, fatty or processed meats, dairy products—especially those produced from cow's milk—are acidifying foods. Food sensitivity tests have emerged due to stomach complaints having become very common. It has to be said at this point that food sensitivity is something we all have—to a greater or lesser degree.

Let's take a quick look at the foods that cause the most food sensitivity:

- Floury foods including oats, wheat, barley, sugar, and rye that contains gluten.

- Dairy products produced from cows; particularly milk, cheese, and yoghurt.

- Food made with yeast such as wine, beer, and bread.

It would be wiser to remove these foods from your food list, not to touch pastry and sweet products, choose those with sourdough when it comes to food containing yeast, and to consume goat's and sheep's milk instead of cow's milk. Even if there may be some sensitivity to these foods, it is usually better to just remove this group. **Indeed, all the foods we constantly mention throughout this book as foods that should be avoided are acidifying foods.** Whether there is sensitivity or not, they should have no place in our diet.

Inflammation of the gut increases either the speed of evacuation causing diarrhea, or slows it down so much that it can cause chronic constipation. Individuals with these complaints should change to a gluten-free, flour-free, and sugar-free diet with no processed animal products, and instead consume plenty of vegetables and good fats. As a result, they will experience a marked change.

Edema in the body is related to problems with gut health. It is accompanied by flatulence and bloating. Foods that cause acidification, especially those that contain gluten, can cause edema in the entire body.

Even if you don't have any gastrointestinal complaints, the situation doesn't change. The foodstuffs listed above exacerbate distant inflammations. Believe me when I say that nearly all diseases progress due to inflammation. Eczema is an inflammation that attacks the skin. Joint pains mean that the joint areas are under attack. The list is very long. Even aging is chronic inflammation.

We should keep a strict distance from these types

of foods, even when it comes to all other diseases that do not involve inflammation.

Nowadays, gluten sensitivity is acknowledged in medical literature, and it has been proven that when a gluten-free diet is applied in treatments for all sorts of diseases—including autism, allergies, arthritis, and depression—it speeds up the healing process. Avoiding gluten reduces inflammation.

We are at the beginning of our knowledge about a healthy diet when it comes to removing gluten from our diets.

Changing to an alkaline diet due to its anti-inflammatory effects is a better option.

Irritable bowel syndrome is closely associated with our emotional states, and **depression** can be one other cause. One of the places where serotonin is produced is the intestines. The production of serotonin declines in damaged intestines that do not function properly.

Stress also creates inflammation of the gut. The functioning of the bowels depends on the **parasympathetic system** (a system of relaxation in the brain that causes relaxation in the entire body) being active. If we are chronically stressed, our **sympathetic system** will be active, not our parasympathetic system. In the event we perceive danger, the sympathetic system transfers the body's energy to the brain, heart, and limbs so that we can flee. Energy is withdrawn from the gut and digestive system. Therefore, it is evident that our parasympathetic system does not work when we are stressed. Delays in mechanical tasks—that can be seen in the evacuation of the bowels or in the production of serotonin in the endocrine system, for instance—are normal when we suffer chronic stress.

In short, if our gut is unhappy, we are unhappy, too!

The gut-brain connection is currently a hot topic. The **vagus nerve** reaches from the gut to the brain and organizes the gut-brain communication. The vagus nerve will only order the gut to work when the brain is free from stress. It is all about the body thinking it is under attack and stopping bowel activity in order to protect us. **If you get stressed easily and, in addition, if you choose to eat bad foods, you will put a lot of pressure on your gut.** As a result, the intestines will also skip serotonin production, causing us to become unhappier and more stressed; thus, it develops into a vicious cycle.

To break this vicious cycle, we have to choose the type of nutrition suitable for our **gut flora.** This brings us back to the same subject we have been discussing at length: alkaline foods.

Microbiota: We Are Not Living for Ourselves, We Are Living for Them

Microbiota is a word you will hear quite frequently. It refers to the bacterial flora in all parts of our bodies, including our guts. The bacteria in our bodies add up to nearly two kilograms. In order for those tiny little things, which can only be seen through a microscope, to amount to two kilograms altogether, they would need to exceed the number of our cells by tenfold. We ought to respect such a great number.

The first organ that should be studied with regards to microbiota is the area with the most bacteria—namely, the gut. The gastrointestinal bacteria are living organisms, too. So, you may be wondering the following: "what do all those bacteria eat and drink inside us?" Similar to other living organisms, they want to be fed a diet suitable for their own environment. Even when we give a simple throat culture sample, it is put in small glass dishes called **petri dishes** containing different nutrients to see which bacteria reproduce. Thus, each bacterium will reproduce on what it prefers and be accordingly identified. **The point I am trying to make from this simple logic is the following: whichever bacteria we wish to increase, we should eat the food they prefer.**

This is not difficult. This is where the perfection of nature kicks in; it whispers to us that whatever food is healthy for us, that food is also healthy for our good bacteria in the gut. If we don't eat suitable nutrients, we cannot reproduce good bacteria. In such a case, the undigested food will be decomposed by other opportunist bacteria, and thus energy will be wasted on them. These opportunists actually take advantage of the necessary bacterial community being absent; as they decompose the bad foods, they increase in numbers. They are, in a way, anticipating to make us ill. The decomposition creates gasses that shouldn't normally be there, and so, we are troubled by flatulence and indigestion.

In a healthy gut, microbiota **symbiosis** is established for a relationship. Symbiosis is about mutual interest, a kind of win-win situation. When we give them what they want, they will also save the bits of food beneficial to us. **Our cooperation with our gut microbiota is so important that protecting it is synonymous with protecting our health.** When the microbiota is healthy, the **intestinal villi** are covered, as if, by a film. The intestinal impermeability is secured by this film. When food particles cannot get inside the intestines to cause inflammation, all inflammation-related illnesses start to heal.

In cases of arthritis, multiple sclerosis, asthma, disorders of the thyroid glands, and many other illnesses that come to mind, inflammation is how many of them emerge.

Recovering gastrointestinal health will reduce complaints of these illnesses.

When the gastrointestinal microbiota protect their own four hundred square meters of space, opportunists cannot reproduce there. Unwanted fungi such as the **candida fungus,** in particular, and other pathogenic bacteria cannot survive when the microbiota are healthy.

I would like to give a special mention to candida here. The candida fungus is the first of the opportunists to reproduce. When candida has multiplied in the gut, it can cause problems with digestion, flatulence, and constipation as well as depression. This means that the production of "the happiness hormone" serotonin is reduced due to the destruction of the intestinal mucosa by candida—also causing a decrease of the precursor of serotonin, the amino acid **L-tryptophan. Candida reproduces particularly when we eat floury and sugary foods containing fructose syrup.** *When fructose from fructose syrup is absorbed by the gastrointestinal tract, it also biochemically takes along the L-tryptophan amino acid, which is the precursor to the serotonin structure. Even when we think we feel happy when we indulge in unhealthy desserts and floury foods, in reality, eating these foods actually make us unhappy.*

You may find the following information interesting. During evolution millions of years ago, our mitochondria were actually bacteria. At the time, there were insufficient nutrients and oxygen to produce energy as there were no plants. Bacteria discovered that they could obtain energy more easily if they lived together in unison. Millions of years later mitochondria evolved from some of those bacteria. In light of their realization then that they needed to unite in order to create a symbiotic structure (considering mutual interest and making each other stronger), we should now understand that we need to create a symbiosis with our gut bacteria and think of their welfare.

Microbiota is a very broad subject. Apart from the

gut, we also have different microbiota in the skin, the nose, the mouth, and the vagina. In the near future, when we truly understand that we need to protect them to protect ourselves, putting on bacterial skin creams or applying special microbiota vaginal gels will become the norm. Perhaps, we will change the concept of bathing to keep our skin young and have baths based on protecting our microbiota. Perhaps, probiotics will be added to all antibiotics. Time will tell.

To sum up, if we are to fight infections caused by bad, external bacteria; if we react very strongly to external factors with disorders such as allergies and suffer from autoimmune diseases such as arthritis and thyroid complaints, we should first regulate the nutrients we put in our gut.

Inflammation Is Inflamm-aging

It is clear that the first source of chronic inflammation is the gut. That much is understood. But why does everything start with inflammation? Inflammation is the body's attempt to correct something it does not like, and it focuses on one specific area and undertakes an attack there. Its purpose is to heal or repair. **But the area it has chosen as target of attack is wrong. When we more closely observe the biochemical modulators of the inflammation or, in other words, at the weapons using inflammation, we discover that they are free radicals.**

- bacterial

- viral

- trauma-induced

- surgery-induced

- cancerous

- allergic

- autoimmune-based

Whatever the reason may be, the formation of a disease at micro level is caused by **an inflammation**. Only people who are one hundred percent healthy have no inflammation.

Of course, the use of inflammation as defence against the bacteria or virus that enter the body—and the use of free radicals as weapons—is good. The purpose is to protect ourselves. In this way, external agents are destroyed. But this is for short-term and healthy inflammations. If we get a cut or have a tooth extracted, it's normal to have inflammation to repair the wound.

Inflammation is like attracting the cell's attention to one area. It is an attempt to solve whatever the problem is at that area. Free radicals, what we call inflammatory modulators, are used for this. When the repair is over, **anti-inflammatory agents** are released to clear away these free radicals. Once it has all been completed, it is the **anti-inflammatory mediators** that do the cleaning up. **They diminish the damage caused** by the free radicals and function as antioxidant mediators.

When inflammation becomes chronic, inflamm-aging speeds up. Unprovoked attacks on the body are reasons for accelerated aging. In the end, aging (for instance, wrinkled-skin) is really chronic inflammation of the skin. **Spots on the skin and the hair going gray are types of inflammation.** We can see that the rate of aging with regards to our appearance is related to our nutrition. The more food we consume containing electrons, or the more anti-inflammatory or antioxidant food we eat, the more we will minimize our inflammation and the rate of our aging. **In conclusion, an alkaline diet containing antioxidants and electrons is, actually, an anti-inflammatory diet.**

The Aging of the Skin and Glycation

Readers of my earlier books will be familiar with **glycation**. But as a quick reminder and in order to give a little knowledge to those who are being introduced to this subject through this book, let's take a closer look at glycation.

Our skin ages because of the cross-link between body proteins and glycose. This means that sugar bonds with the **collagen** protein causing **glycation**. There is no return from this bonding. The result of the bonding is that collagen loses its suppleness, slackens, and droops. The underlying cause of skin problems, even cellulite, is glycation. Moreover, glycation affects the eyes and can even lead to cataracts. The consequence of glycation is the formation of **advanced glycation endproducts (AGEs).** AGEs play an active role in nearly all age-related illnesses.

Glycation can be slowed down through an alkaline diet. However, after the cross-link between body proteins and glycose occurs, there is no going back.

Do not forget that all food that has been cooked or fried at high temperature is a store for AGEs, which are full of protons. The more you eat this kind of food, the sooner you will age!

Fattening Around the Waistline

Fat around the waistline causes inflammation and therefore illnesses. Inflammation causes inflammatory substances to be formed in the fatty tissues, and from there they spread to the rest of the body. **These substances create their own inflammation wherever they go.** If there is already chronic disease in the body spreading through inflammation, the substances from fat around the waistline will exacerbate the symptoms of that illness.

While there are no tests that make it possible to measure that the fat around the waistline increases all sorts of complaints such as heart problems, rheumatism, breast cysts, and fibromyalgia, it is a fact. The most efficient way of losing this fat is to control your evening meals.

It is up to us to avoid fattening of the upper body, which keeps the whole body in a sort of chronically ill state, producing unwanted hormones and overworking the endocrine organ. Below are some simple clues. These recommendations can also be noted as the healthiest way to lose weight.

How to Lose Belly Fat

- The quickest way to lose weight around the waist is to have your dinner before 5 p.m. If you have nothing else but herbal tea and water after that time, you will lose weight much faster. You can have a hearty dinner before 5 p.m.

- If dinner is left until after 5 p.m., have it as early as possible. Preferably, the evening meal should consist of vegetables. As long as you eat vegetables, there is no limit to the amount.

- If you insist on having something else besides vegetables for dinner, this can be fish, grilled meat, turkey, or chicken. You should also eat at least three times more salad and vegetables than these animal proteins.

- Dairy products, dried fruit and nuts, floury foods, pulses, and fruit are not appropriate for the evening meal and thereafter. These products should not be consumed after 5 p.m.

- If you don't have your dinner earlier and in a smaller portion, you will not achieve weight loss (and maintain it) simply by limiting your calorie intake throughout the day.

- All kinds of floury foods, sweet foods, processed meat, dairy products from cow's milk, sugary soft drinks, alcohol, and preprepared sauces should not be consumed. Even those with few calories, i.e., diet food, make the body acidic and will cause weight gain.

- All kinds and any amount of raw or lightly cooked vegetables, spices, fatty seeds (e.g. linseeds and nigella seeds), oily nuts (e.g. walnuts and almonds), raw fruit, pulses, and fish can be eaten throughout the day. Once a week, you can eat red meat; once a day, an egg as well as one portion of milk, cheese, or yogurt from sheep's, goat's, or buffalo's milk.

- No floury foods are acceptable. Especially, wheat, barley, rye, and oats that contain gluten should not be eaten. No products containing sugar are acceptable.

Fibromyalgia: Unending Muscle Pain for No Apparent Reason

Fibromyalgia is a widespread disorder that is quite

painful and disturbing. Usually, sufferers of this condition are unable to find a cure. **In taking a microscopic look at fibromyalgia, we observe that there is some kind of inflammation of the muscles, and that the muscles cannot relax but stay hard and taut.** Though many different treatment types are recommended, particularly for back pain, they may not produce a complete cure.

When the tissue and muscles of fibromyalgia patients are tested, we see an overload of lactic acid. **Don't forget that lactic acid uses the inefficient Plan B rather than Plan A for energy production.** We observe that in fibromyalgia, the mitochondria of the painful muscles do not work properly and cannot produce Plan A energy.

Muscles that produce energy without oxygen produce lactic acid from glucose. This yields only very little ATP, whereas energy is needed for the muscles to relax. We need energy both for our muscles to contract and to relax. For instance, **rigor mortis**, the stiffening of the body in death, is the inability of the muscles to relax due to lack of energy. Another example can be seen in constipation—usually accompanying fibromyalgia—when mitochondria in the intestinal muscles are unable to produce enough energy.

The lactic acid collecting in the muscles is also the reason for muscle pains in the back. **Recommendations to minimize lactic acid and increase mitochondrial energy would be useful in the treatment of** fibromyalgia.

For the body to change from a Plan A to Plan B energy model, there must be either insufficient oxygen, or the mitochondria must be damaged by free radicals, thus, preventing them from working properly. **To overcome breathing problems caused by a nose deviation or sleep apnea, for instance, fibromyalgia sufferers can find relief in relaxation and breathing exercises.** Supporting the energy production of the mitochondria will also reduce their complaints.

Chronic Fatigue Syndrome: Waking Up Exhausted Every Morning

Chronic fatigue syndrome can, like fibromyalgia, arise due to mitochondria or energy production being insufficient. Sometimes there are hormonal reasons; the **burnout syndrome** that occurs when the adrenal gland is overworked by our hormones can also cause chronic fatigue. Yet, in any case, the problem is the inadequate energy production of the mitochondria at the cellular level. For our body to produce more energy, it needs more oxygen. Energy is produced more easily and in greater amounts in the body where there is oxygen.

A good way to approach chronic fatigue syndrome is to view it as mitochondrial fatigue. To minimize mitochondrial fatigue, the production of oxygen-based energy should be increased; this would be beneficial for all the diseases I have so far mentioned. In order to produce high energy, electrons and oxygen need to be transported to the mitochondria. This is where the blood's pH value becomes important.

Oxygen is transported by the blood, which must always be alkaline. The blood maintains its pH in the narrow gap of 7.35-7.45. If our blood pH falls from 7.45 to 7.35 and becomes 0.1 less alkaline, though it may seem like an insignificant difference, it will have a very important effect. This tiny difference decreases the blood's **capacity to transport oxygen**. The capacity might fall by thirty percent—a decrease in oxygen capacity that is almost the same as not taking one in three breaths.

As it is vitally important, the blood will always maintain its pH within this narrow scope. The pH value must not move more than 0.1 points. This is normal, and anything else cannot maintain life. The body has many mechanisms to preserve this state. These precautions are called the **acid-base buffer system**. It is true that the pH of blood, whatever we do and despite all bad nutritional and life choices, will not exceed the limits. But even the tiny 0.1 percent change it allows itself can change the blood's oxygen capacity by thirty percent. When this becomes chronic, it becomes a big problem. The blood that delivers oxygen to the furthest cell of the entire body will decrease by one-third.

The amount of blood is also important, because it transports oxygen. We know that people with chronic anaemia (blood deficiency) complain of tiredness.

When there is only a little blood, transportation of oxygen is also little, and from a little oxygen only a little energy is produced, and the result is tiredness. Thus, anaemia should be treated.

When the blood pH moves a tiny fraction towards acidity, it causes the free radicals to increase, which also increases the protons. Let's remember that pH in any kind of fluid (in this case blood) is a proton charge. When we feed mitochondria with poor food from negatively charged electrons (-), positively charged protons (+) fill up the surroundings, and the pH alkaline value in the cell decreases. In fact, the higher the alkaline value, the more oxygen there is.

In conclusion, one of the basic negative effects of food that acidifies the blood is that it lowers the body's oxygen uptake. Eating acidifying food suffocates us little by little. And, this ultimately leads to cancer.

Cancer: How Scared Should We Be?

A cancer cell is simply a cell that works without mitochondria. **The cancer cell uses Plan B to produce energy rather than Plan A.** The more it does this, the more the lactic acid in it increases and the median pH value drifts even more towards acidity. When acidification increases, oxygen cannot be harbored there. Everything moves even further towards obtaining anaerobic energy. Dr Otto Warburg received a Nobel prize for having discovered that the cancer cell produced anaerobic energy. For this reason, whenever a cell produces anaerobic energy, it is medically known as the Warburg effect. The Warburg effect is found in all cancers.

Glucose, which is suitable for anaerobic energy, is the fuel of the Warburg effect. It is the cheap fuel of Plan B. Also, fats are of no benefit to the cancer cells. Since the mitochondria are not working, and there is little oxygen, the only place for the cell to produce energy is the cytoplasm—where it produces a little anaerobic energy with glucose. **Of course, this small amount of energy, besides not being sufficient for any work, is also not enough to prevent the mitochondria from being damaged nor to repair them.**

If the immunity cells do not see this "damaged" cell and destroy it, or if the cell does not decide to commit suicide, these cells will not die but continue to reproduce. Cancer cells are cells with the thickest cell membranes due to acidification. The membranes have become so thick that they have been surrounded by a substance called **fibrin**.

In this membrane thickened with fibrin, the healthy electrical voltage changes. The normal number of negative (-) charges decreases (i.e., the electrons) and the plus (+) charges (i.e., the free radicals, or protons) increase and change the voltage. **When the electrical current inside and outside the cell changes, the connection between this cell and the other cells weakens.**

The voltage in the membranes of cancer cells is

lower than before. When the membranes become rigid, the electrical current passing through the membrane decreases. The unsaturated fatty lipids in the membrane change into a fully-saturated fatty structure; from being a thin and liquid fat such as oil, they become solid as margarine. The electrons flowing over these membranes have decreased.

As the electrons decrease, the vibration of the atoms also decreases. It is the number of electrons surrounding the atoms that make them vibrate. Membrane vibration and voltage is an important subject, because it is these electrical and vibrational signals that enable the cells to identify one another and work in harmony, even from a long distance, and be informed. **This is a quantum method of communication**; it takes place over electromagnetic areas.

The immunity detectors can very easily miss it when the cancer cell loses its voltage and vibration. Just as it is with insulin resistance that the lock and the insulin in the rigid membranes don't recognize one another, it also becomes difficult for the body to recognize the membrane of the cancer cell; therefore, it becomes foreign to the body.

Moreover, the latest chemotherapies have treatment methods by which they first get rid of the cancer cell's thick outer membrane in order for the medication to reach inside the cell more swiftly. For the thick shell to get thinner, once again, an alkaline diet is necessary. Protecting the decreasing good, unsaturated fat on the membrane by using vegetables to provide electrons against the free radicals makes good sense in the support of cancer treatment.

Of course, modern medical treatment is necessary as well as diet. What I want to explain here is not the frightfulness of the disease, but the simplicity of it. Our task is simple. **To eat healthy alkaline food that increases our quantum energy and to live a life that sustains this.** The saying "*you are what you eat*" makes sense.

The relationship between cancer and genetics is frequently debated. Of course, each of us have a code in our genes. These codes are **mute/turned off**. For them to remain turned off, the DNA mustn't be damaged. But by not adhering to an alkaline diet and exposing our body to protons, or rather free radicals, the DNA may eventually get damaged; therefore, the genes will become vocal, turn on the switch, and cause illness. The biggest source of free radicals, meanwhile, is badly functioning mitochondria. Mitochondria are now the focus for an early cancer diagnosis and to develop treatment.

Other diseases related to insufficient energy production by the mitochondria are listed below.

In the muscles:

- weakness

- cramps
- lack of endurance while exercising
- getting tired quickly
- muscle slackness

In the brain:

- autism
- slowed development
- migraine
- stroke

In the liver:

- non-alcohol related fatty liver disease

In the heart:

- heart failure

All these diseases manifest in our bodies when mitochondria do not produce enough energy. In fact, in every illness that entails cell damage, it is a question of engine and fuel. Now that we have learned the problems with our engines, let's choose the correct fuel.

Chapter 5:

Quantum Electronic Eating...

The Name is Really Cool!

Why quantum? Because, nutritional science is explained in terms of the subatomic world. Why electronic? Because, we have little organic batteries that work by producing bioelectric energy with electrons, the heroes of the subatomic world.

We are not simple living organisms. If we accept we are the most superior of creatures, it is obvious that we accept, technically, we have the most superior qualities. Science permitting, this complex structure of ours will be revealed (in the future) in the finest detail. For the moment, however, the quantum biology approach is the best in explaining our uniqueness. This means, we must update the old-style elementary perceptions.

What Is Food, And What Is Not?

The fact that something is called **"food"** does not necessarily mean that it is actually food. A great many things filling the supermarket shelves as food are, in fact, rubbish for the body. They are not food but the opposite, **"anti-foods."** They are not nutrients; they are **"anti-nutrients."** To call something food, it must evidently fit the methods for obtaining our energy and quantum biology, which are the phases of our mitochondria's energy cycles.

- Food must suit the mitochondria!

- Food must feed the cell and mitochondrion, not the stomach!

- Feed your mitochondrion, not your stomach!

The whole energy production system in the mitochondria occurs with electrons and protons, the tiny subatomic particles. Anything to the contrary is out of the question. In that case, where electrons and protons are mentioned, we ought to use the term quantum; furthermore, we should know that this biology is now **quantum biology**, and its rules have to be obeyed.

The behavior patterns of our electrons display quantum characteristics. This quantum behavior is in the micro-basis of all metabolic events including thinking, sleeping, producing energy, and intercellular communication.

The quantum world is rather strange next to the

rules of Newtonian physics. After all, Newtonian physics cannot explain to us most of the phenomena in the body. For instance, we know that faster-than-light intercellular communication or the conscience exists, but we cannot show their location in the brain. The day is near when answers will be given to these kind of questions. However, for now, we can make our argument up to the following point: if we eat in accordance with quantum biology, our awareness will increase. The state of enlightenment, awareness, and higher consciousness are fundamental in being an **"upgraded person."**

Thus, we will rise to the top in evolution.

If we want our body cells to be **"upgraded"** in this way, the quantum properties of our diets and lifestyles need to be enhanced. We owe our quantum properties to our electrons, which are present in everything that is matter—more in some substances and less in others.

The things we look for in food must have the quality to increase electrons. Our understanding of health, therefore, must be to increase the electrons in the body. **I claim that our life is as long as our electrons.** In that case, nutrition can be reduced to knowing about the sources of our electrons.

Plants: The Miracle Secret on the Path to Eternal Life

- vegetables
- fruit

- spices

- seeds

- pulses

- nuts

All of the above food items come into the plant group. All plants grow by performing photosynthesis; they materialize the sunlight as fruit, leaves, or roots.

Photosynthesis is **endergonic**; that is, it is an event where energy is absorbed. Energy production in our mitochondria is the complete opposite to photosynthesis. It is an **exergonic** reaction, in which energy is released. The sources that release the highest energy, so that we may produce a lot of energy, must be our food. All foods that come to mind under the heading of "plants" are considered healthy, because they are sources that provide the highest energy for electrons. However, it must not be forgotten that **plants have the most electrons** when they are raw and fresh.

Is It Healthy to Cook Them?

The way healthy food is consumed also determines the amount of electrons. The reason why vegetables are beneficial is because they contain vitamins, minerals, plant proteins, and antioxidants. However, these benefits will decrease with cooking. First of all, all types of vegetables are beneficial. **In terms of the quality as an antioxidant, the deeper the color of the vegetable,** the greater its capacity to remove free radicals.

Antioxidants are high in all plants, but **purple vegetables and fruit have the highest ORAC (oxygen radical absorbance capacity).** Unfortunately, though, cooking destroys almost more than half of the antioxidants.

In green vegetables, one can find chlorophyll, which is the plant's blood. It is almost the same as the hemoglobin in our blood. It gives us the oxygen it obtains from the plant. Therefore, to eat chlorophyll is like breathing oxygen. Chlorophyll also contains iron and magnesium. **Again, cooking destroys chlorophyll**.

Vegetables have enzymes. In fact, plants facilitate their digestion with their own enzymes; they do not use a lot of the body's enzymes—some of which are produced in the pancreas to help us digest our food. Thus, plants do not tire the pancreas. Furthermore, enzymes do not merely help digestion, they do much more. For instance, remember what I discussed about cancer cells: they cover their walls with a thick web in order to hide from the immune system. If the enzymes in the body penetrate through this web, the immune system can catch the cancerous cell and destroy it. **But unfortunately, because we consume so much food of animal origin, our enzymes' sole job becomes digesting these foods.** On the contrary, if we eat mainly vegetables—especially raw vegetables—they will digest themselves with their own enzymes and not put a strain on the pancreas.

Cooking vegetables reduces their water content.

Yet, that water contains very valuable minerals. These minerals cannot be produced in the body; we have to be get them externally—through food. Vegetables obtain minerals from the earth and we obtain them from vegetables. Selenium, magnesium, potassium, and boron are some of the minerals we obtain from vegetables. There are few minerals that can be found in foods of animal origin.

Cooking vegetables reduces the protein they contain.

Yet, there is plant protein in all vegetables, and it is very beneficial.

Cooking vegetables reduces the vitamin value by half.

Cooking vegetables at high heat, or frying them, turns them into almost useless rubbish. Don't forget, if we fry broccoli even, it will become a storage of harmful free radicals. Furthermore, when vegetables, such as purslane, containing good fatty acids (omega-3) are cooked, the fatty acids (of this type) oxidize and are of no benefit.

Cooking harms the plants' atomic structure.

In order to be healthy, we need electrons more than anything. And it is raw vegetables that store electrons, which are able to remedy all health-related maladies. General statements, such as "cooking causes a loss of vitamins and minerals," are, in fact, insufficient in explaining the situation. What does need to be said, however, is that electrons decrease with cooking.

I won't even go into the damage of methods such as microwave ovens, which change the vegetable's atomic structure without recourse. But, contact with heat in any way will destroy the effectiveness of the plants.

Even the most innocuous cooking methods, such as steaming and boiling, will reduce the solar energy inside plants and vegetables.

If foods are raw, they carry more sunlight; more photon energy; more electrons; more antioxidants; and more alkaline properties. The terms here are all the same.

But getting back to the topic of color, we must care about the colors of plants. Let's take a quick look below to find out why.

Eat with the Rainbow

All **green-leaved vegetables** contain a large amount of chlorophyll. Chlorophyll is the plants' little organ that absorbs the sunlight. The light absorbed by chlorophyll will be stored in the plant's leaves, roots, and fruit as electrons. All colors of vegetables are good. However, the number of stored electrons can change according to the color of the plant.

We know from our simple high school knowledge

of physics that when sunlight passes through a prism, it splits into seven different colors. These seven colors have different wavelengths. While sunlight in red has the least energy but the longest wavelength, the light in purple has the highest energy but the shortest wavelength. Wavelength and energy are opposite to each other. When the wavelength shortens, energy increases. The reason for the increased energy is that the matter's atoms have more electrons. **And so, we can easily make the following deduction: there are more electrons in purple foods.**

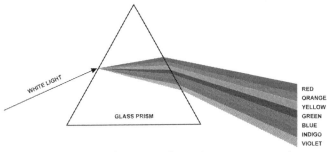

Figure 8: When light passes through a prism, it splits into seven colors.

Due to their high antioxidant properties, the benefits of purple vegetables and fruits to health are often mentioned in the press. We should by now understand that the term antioxidants, or the special names for antioxidants such as **polyphenol** and **resveratrol**, actually means there is an abundance of electrons. Let us recap once again.

- If electrons are abundant, antioxidants are abundant, too.
- Electrons are antioxidant.
- Electrons are alkaline.

Which foods are purple?

- purple grapes

- beetroot

- blueberries

- red turnips

- red cabbage

- eggplants

- pomegranates

- plums

- blackberries

- red onions

For instance, the proportion of electrons in a beetroot is so great that it increases the oxygen-carrying capacity of our body. Eggplant skins contain so many electrons that creams made from them have begun to be used in the treatment of skin cancer. (Cancer is the disease with the greatest free radical damage.)

In fact, rather than focusing on one or two

examples, it would be more correct to think of our system holistically. If you hear that a food is good for one disease, you should know that it will also be good for all other diseases. **This is because a cell is a cell. Something that is good for one is good for them all.** All cells use the same system in basic energy production, repair, and in methods for cleaning up rubbish. The difference arises from the fact that cells perform different duties depending on the organ in which they reside. **Cells perform different duties, but the operating system is the same.**

Under the heading of plants, every color of vegetable, fruit, or even flowers can be put on the list of items that should be eaten. They are all good. What is important is that they should be close to their natural forms. **Of course, it is better if they are freshly harvested.** The best are those found in local farmers' markets. But, even if we have to buy from the neighborhood greengrocer, plants are far superior to processed foods.

For those who are concerned about agricultural pesticides and prefer not to eat the skins, I have some sad news; unfortunately, the **essential high concentration of electrons is in the skins.** For instance, it is good to eat the whole lemon, chopping it with its skin and not just to squeeze the lemon and drink the juice. **This habit of peeling the skin to eat must change.** People must realize that to eat lemons, apples, eggplants, watermelons, and so on, with the skin is much better. In fact, the skins and seeds are even better than the inside of the plant.

Kernels and Seeds

Kernels and seeds carry the plant's growth information inside them. We know that matter is actually compressed energy. But, the latest point science has reached is that energy is information. Everything in the universe is different versions of information.

What we should know is that it is primarily the seeds that have the plant's **information**. Nigella, sesame, linseed, and all the tiny little seeds you can think of are particles of compressed electrons, energy, and information. The seeds and the shoots formed from these seeds are intelligent ways of obtaining the universe's energy. Pulses, such as lentils and beans, are also types of seeds. **Inside seeds, there are good fats that give concentrated energy to the plant, because the plant will grow and develop taking nourishment from these seeds. Seeds are important in terms of the fat they carry.**

It is far more beneficial to eat them by germinating them—to revive them and bring to light the information inside them. The shoots of pulses are better than the pulses themselves.

Nuts and Spices

Walnuts, almonds, and hazelnuts, and others in the nut

group, are ultimately plants as well. They are good electron donors if they are fresh and raw. The fats of nuts are important as a source of electrons.

Spices, however, are good just because they are plants. A kind of "concentrated plant," spices have such a high antioxidant property that we know turmeric for its anti-tumor qualities and cinnamon for its effect on diabetes. They have even begun to be given as injections instead of just being consumed orally. They are being used as complementary medicine to conventional treatments for various diseases that are chronic inflammatory or tumor-related. Do not think of this information as **"nonmedical."** Conventional treatments will still continue. However, the ever-increasing number of studies and their results is making physicians change from synthetic drugs to those obtained from biological substances.

How Much Sunlight Is Latent in the Food You Eat?

The inclusion of enzymes, minerals, vitamins, and fiber in vegetables have macro-level benefits. We constantly hear this. **However, the most fundamental benefit is in their electron, or rather their antioxidant, capacities.** There are different units of measurement for antioxidant capacity. The measurement of a plant's antioxidant capacity is shown with ORAC (oxygen radical absorbance capacity). The ORAC value shows the capacity of a substance to destroy its free radicals. It is a substance's capacity to give electrons to free radicals.

Plants, vegetables, fruit, spices, and nuts can be listed in their own groups in terms of their ORAC value. The higher the ORAC value the better. The ORAC value can be adopted in everyday speech as the **rust-removing value**. If we do not want to rust, we must pursue the high ORAC value in foods. Of course, the ORAC value in fresh plants cannot be compared with that in processed products.

ORAC shows the electron value in plants. Electrons come from photons, and photons come from light. **ORAC is ultimately the amount of sunlight hidden inside the plant**. It is not difficult to understand that the ORAC value is high in colored vegetables, fruits, and spices where there is a large concentration of electrons.

Food	Consumption Preference	ORAC Value (100 Grams)
sumac bran	raw	300,900
wild marjoram	dried	165,712
cinnamon	powder	143,264
thyme	dried	137,720
rosemary	dried	112,200

clove	powder	111,490
sage	ground	98,714
rosehip	raw	96,150
parsley	dried	68,417
basil	dried	56,685
cumin	powder	47,600
turmeric	powder	44,776
sage	fresh	32,004
thyme	fresh	27,426
oregano	fresh	27,297
curry	powder	24,980
paprika	powder	21,827
raspberry	raw	19,220
walnut (pecan)	raw	17,524
ginger root	raw	14,840
mint	raw	13,978
caper	raw	13,750
walnut	raw	13,057

black pepper	powder	10,205
blueberry	raw	9,621
pear	dried	9,496
cornelian cherry	raw	8,888
plum	dried	7,880

The **ORP (oxidation reduction potential)** value is generally used for fluids and, as with ORAC, is used to explain in a similar way the amount of electrons in the fluids we drink and air we breathe. The ORP value is expressed as plus (+) or minus (-) charges. Since the minus (-) value shows the electron charge and the plus (+) value shows the proton charge, the more minuses (-) the ORP value has, the more electrons there are in that fluid. It means that the fluid is antioxidant and alkaline. It is not difficult to see that the fluid with a plus (+) ORP value will be an acidified fluid full of protons, containing free radicals.

Vegetable juices have a high negative ORP value. Alkaline drinking water has a negative ORP value. Fruit juices with little sugar also have a negative ORP value. However, in drinks such as alcohol, coffee, sodas, and processed fluids like synthetic fruit juices, the ORP value is positive. We should know that we will end up wasting our minus value electrons in order to destroy the plus ORP values in these liquids that we drink.

We are always reading about the detrimental effects of these types of drinks. Well, this is the real damage. There are no antioxidant electrons in them, only free radicals. When we look at the pH in sodas such as cola, we see that it is below 7. These drinks are acidic and their plus (+) proton values are in excess. Drinks with a negative ORP value must be favored.

In order to preserve their true capacities, foods with good ORP and ORAC values should not be processed. In processed foods, these values rapidly diminish. You probably already know about the harms of packaged supermarket products—which have been written about everywhere, but the cooking methods you are accustomed to at home are no longer acceptable either. **The right step to take is to obtain nutrients in the most natural state possible.**

Fats: Friend or Foe?

The other fundamental need in our diets is good fats. They protect the membranes of cells. Well, are fats friend or foe? Fats are one of the two most important issues in nutrition. While foods rich in electrons are the first and more important subject, fats are second in importance.

First of all, we must know that all cells on the outside and all the organelles such as the nucleus, mitochondria, and ribosome inside them, are separated from each other by membranes. The organelles and cells protect themselves thanks to the membranes. This is because membranes have selective permeability, and special systems open and close to prevent the passage of anything harmful to them. These membranes have to be very thin and pliable. Thinness, pliancy, and durability are features provided by the fats in the membrane structure.

If they did not have these features, the cell membranes would lose their permeability, electric voltage, vibrations, and their ability to obey the orders of hormones. **If we remember that in each of the forty billion cells there are thousands of mitochondria, we will grasp that it is even more important that the mitochondrial membranes are protected.**

One must always remember the following point: the mitochondrial membrane is the place where energy is obtained. In case of an inadequacy in generating energy, the mitochondrion will suffer free radical damage, causing the membrane to become oxidized—which, in turn, will decrease energy further. If there is no energy, the mitochondrion will be unable to do its task. **If there is no energy, the diseased cell will not be able to repair itself.** We understand this simple logic.

There are unsaturated fats on the membranes—the targets of free radicals. These unsaturated fats are in a position to donate their electrons. The reason they are the first target of attack in free radical damage is the fact that oxidization of these membrane-fats is easier. In that case, replacing the unsaturated fats that free radicals will take from the membranes is a sufficient way to repair the membranes. Well, it is here that the importance of eating **good fats** becomes evident.

Good fat is essential to repair the membrane lipids!

As much as the amount of unsaturated fat on the membrane is connected to the pliancy and thinness of the membrane, it is also related to the electrical conductivity. Oxidation of the membrane lipids changes the electric voltage of the membranes.

The voltage on the membrane is necessary,

- first, for ATP production.

- second, for the cells to recognize each other.

The speed of the ability to make contact is related to the membrane voltage. **The conduction speed in the brain and nervous system, in particular, depend entirely on the voltage of the cell membranes being at the required level.** The membranes of brain cells have the most fat. The most mitochondria are in the cells of the brain. This is because fast conduction and high energy are needed.

- third, for the cells to perform their duties.

Among their tasks are taking in the nutrients, taking out the rubbish, producing protein, renewing the worn-out parts, and remedying diseases.

In that case, repairing the cell must start first from

the mitochondria and membranes. Consuming good fats is important in order to give electrons to these membranes.

Which Fats Are Healthy?

There is confusion as to which fats are good and which are bad. Let me try to clarify this here. Readers of my first two books know the subject, so this will be review for them. And those of you who are beginning the whole subject of alkaline and quantum eating from this book should learn this.

Good Fats	Where They Are Found	Benefits
omega-3	fish: salmon, tuna, anchovy, and mackerel vegetables: linseed, kiwi, purslane, walnuts, almonds, hazelnuts, and nigella seeds	protects from disease; prevents depression
coconut oil	coconuts	speeds up metabolism; reduces physical fatigue; slows

		brain damage connected to alzheimer's
seed oils	linseeds, sesame, almonds, hazelnuts, walnuts, nigella, sunflower, pumpkin	stores omega-3; contains calcium and magnesium
butter	animals	protects the intestine; rapidly converts to energy
other good fats	olive oil, sesame oil, nigella oil, linseed oil, the oils of nuts (e.g., walnuts, almonds, and hazelnuts), fish oil, krill oil	they act like all other good fats.

The Lengths of Fats: the Short, Medium, and Long

Fats display chemical differences and are separated into three groups according to the length of their chain: the long-chain, medium-chain, and short-chain. We can give butter as an example of the short-chain fatty acids. And we can consider coconut oil as one of the medium-chain fatty acids. The best known long-chain fat is margarine.

We can compare long-chain fatty acids and medium-chain fatty acids in this way:

✓ When long-chain fatty acids are absorbed from the intestine, they are transported by the lymph to the liver: medium-chain fatty acids are not transported by the lymph but rather directly, more speedily to the liver by the blood.

✓ When long-chain fatty acids (with more than 20 carbons) enter the mitochondria to be burnt in the liver, they are transported with carnitine—a fatty acid carrier. Those in the medium-chain (with less than 20 carbons) enter the mitochondria quickly without carnitine.

✓ Long-chain fats first become medium-chain in a special micro-particle called peroxisome. Medium-chain fats do not lose time in peroxisome.

✓ In one gram of long-chain fats, there are nine calories. In one gram of medium-chain fats, there are 8.3 calories; they have ten percent less calories.

✓ Long-chain fats require storing. Medium-chain fats prefer to be burnt instead of being stored.

✓ Long-chain fats form their ketone bodies later. Medium-chain fats can form ketone bodies immediately.

✓ It takes a long time for long-chain fats to convert to energy for the brain and muscle. The conversion of medium-chain fats to energy in the brain and muscle is very quick.

✓ Biotin and vitamin B12 are needed to burn long-chain fats. They are more difficult to burn with a vitamin B12 deficiency. (This means that if we want to dissolve stomach fat, we must not neglect our vitamin B12. All our stored fats are long-chain.) Medium-chain fats are directly absorbed without the need for vitamin B12. They are even used in enhancing the athlete's performance.

It is clear that we produce good quality energy from the short- and medium-chain fats in our diet. We need to consume plenty of these fats without hesitation.

Even if we have perfectly working mitochondria, while we produce 36 ATP from one sugar molecule, we produce 129 ATP from one fatty acid.

In addition, I must mention the importance of short-chain fatty acids in keeping the intestine healthy. Short-chain fats normally produce a high level of healthy probiotics necessary in the gut flora. The raw materials for this are the fibers of the foods that have not been digested. Fiber nutrients provide the raw material to produce short-chain fat for the good bacteria in the gut. Vegetables are the source of these fibers, which come from the small intestine without being digested. These are turned into short-chain fatty acids by the bacteria in the large intestine. These short-chain fatty acids ensure both impermeability of the gut, and they also send the signal of fullness to the brain.

They understand that your gut, not your stomach, is full!

The signal of fullness is very much related to having a sufficient number of good bacteria in our gut. We must increase eating fibers. We must add butter, a short-chain fat, to our diet for the health of our gut.

Short-chain fats also have similar advantages to those of the medium-chain. They protect the gall bladder. When they are absorbed by the intestine, they do not need to be absorbed by bile acids such as the long-chain fatty acids; therefore, it makes sense to use them in gall bladder-related problems.

Leptin, the fullness-hormone, gives the signal that we're full. Good fats increase the leptin hormone. Let me share with you some little-known medical knowledge: the hormone leptin works like the electron-meter of the hypothalamus area of the brain. If there is a lot of energy from the electrons, leptin tells us we are full. However, when we eat food that has few electrons, leptin will not give the signal of fullness. Since an abundance of electrons means an abundance of minus (-) charges, then the positive (-) charges in people who eat badly and put on weight are low. Thus, obese people are positively (+) charged.

The Way to Shine: Biophotons and Fats

If I were to tell you that the fats in your cell membranes could also hold sunlight, would this seem strange?

Cells can hold light by means of the membranes, and even our DNA itself can do this job. Science has proven this. This state, called **biophoton emission**, can be measured spectrophotometrically.

We also need sunlight as much as plants. This is why it is not surprising that as we go towards the poles, where there is little sun, the sources of food shift towards cold-water sea fish with omega-3 to balance this need. From this point of view, because animals also need the sun, it is logical that fish living devoid of light in the depths of the cold seas contain more omega-3. **When evaluated in this way, it can be deduced that omega-3 oils can convert light from the photon-state to the electron-state and retain it.**

While we are on the subject of the sun again, let's

also take a look at vitamin D.

To Catch the Sun: Vitamin D and Oils

Does the amount of vitamin D in our bodies show our capacity to keep sunlight inside us? The vitamin D synthesis in our skin—or its retention of sun rays with the pigment melanin—is a kind of quantum biological chain of events.

The importance of vitamin D has been emphasized a great deal. However, it would be questionable to think that this vitamin merely concerns the calcium-bone metabolism. Vitamin D is necessary to eliminate deficiencies in every illness; for instance, it helps to prevent cancer and reduce vigorous allergic reactions.

Why is vitamin D deficiency so common, then? Despite the fact that almost everyone sunbathes, be it an adult or child, vitamin D is at a low level. Here, we must look at the big picture again. If we utilize our skin to benefit from the sun, we must increase the skin's light-retentiveness with a diet of good fats and plenty of electrons. Our vitamin D deficiency increases when our cells have difficulty in absorbing light. **The fact that the sun today produces more skin cancer and sunspots compared to the past can also be linked to this phenomenon.**

For light to be healthily absorbed, the skin needs cell membranes that can absorb the light so that it can pass through the surface of the skin. **In that case, even if it**

is solely to avoid sunspots, we should nourish the skin with oil and electrons as well as sun protection on hot days. In my opinion, the fact that we have little light is evident from low levels of vitamin D, and electron and oil supplements are needed as much as a vitamin D supplement. If vitamin D and omega-3 supplements are necessary, they must be arranged by a physician.

In order to increase levels of vitamin D, the customary animal foods of the dairy group have given way to foods that can be found as plants with good fats and seeds, such as sesame.

Animal Foods: Should They Be Completely Cut Out?

I frequently encounter this question. Let's find the answer together. Animal-based foods are foods from which we **indirectly** take in the sun. While we **directly** take in the sun when we eat plant-based foods, this process is not direct when we eat animal-based foods.

Consequently, the journey in our body of animal proteins is also different from that of vegetables. During this journey, our body has to exert much effort. I have already discussed this subject in detail in my previous books. But in order to inform new readers, here is a quick summary.

The first eleven reasons why animal proteins are undesirable are as follows:

    1. Too much stomach acid is required to digest

animal proteins.

2. Digestion of animal protein exhausts the pancreas.

3. Digestion of animal protein makes us lose electrons.

4. There is a high risk of animal proteins increasing inflammation.

5. Animal proteins decompose in the intestine.

6. It is extremely likely that animal proteins contain hormones.

7. Animal proteins increase ammonia.

8. Animal proteins speed up aging—which can lead to high cholesterol, cancer, osteoporosis, and kidney diseases.

9. Animal proteins acidify the body.

10. Animal proteins are a proton (+) store.

11. Animal proteins are full of saturated fats.

How much protein should be taken?

Under these circumstances, the question of how much animal protein we need for a healthy life immediately arises? The answer is that red meat can be eaten one to two times a week:

- If it is well chewed.

- If it is not combined with carbohydrates.

- If four times the amount of raw vegetables are eaten with it.

- If the source of protein is a naturally grazing animal.

When we look at it in terms of the health of the mitochondria, there are amino acids called **arginine**, **methionine**, and **cysteine** in animal proteins.

- Eating liver is a good source of methionine.

- Eggs and cheese curd are the best sources of cysteine.

- Bone broth is important for regenerating the skin and joints, and for gut health and immunity.

- Of course, fish should be preferred for their omega-3.

We can also add a small amount of turkey, organic lamb, and veal; as well as dairy products from goats, sheep, and water buffaloes to this group. However, no more than the required amount should be eaten because of the damages mentioned above. **There are plenty of vegetable protein sources. The fear of being without protein in attempts to eat healthily is unfounded.**

Oxygen and Diet

For healthy mitochondria, apart from food containing electrons, our main basic need is oxygen. Without oxygen, the fire won't burn. Without oxygen, we would lose our lives within a few minutes. The importance of oxygen lies in the fact that without it we cannot produce energy. Remember that our evolution and our being superior to other creatures are connected to our ability to have a great number of mitochondria. A lot of mitochondria means a lot of energy.

With a lot of energy, we can also do a lot of work. Again, if we get ill, we can use this energy for repair. We know that we benefit from electrons in energy production in the mitochondria. Whatever we eat, food will eventually convert into ATP with the burning of electrons with oxygen. **The energy model obtained with oxygen is productive.** Animals and humans use this efficient energy production model. Energy production without oxygen is inefficient. This is used by primitive organisms, anaerobic bacteria, and single-celled organisms.

Oxygen is necessary to burn foods. This means that to be able to transport oxygen to every part of the body for energy is a vital task—which is undertaken by the veins. Blood is the vehicle that transports oxygen from the lungs and carries it to all remote corners of the body. This is done by the blood's "assistants"—the **erythrocytes**, or **red corpuscles**. In some cases, the oxygen transported by the blood increases, and in some cases it lessens.

Below are situations when the oxygen in the blood diminishes:

- smoking cigarettes

- exposure to air pollution

- lung diseases

- nose deviation

- sleep apnea

- allergy-related nose congestion

- holding of the breath for psychological reasons

These are macro-reasons. The diminishing of the oxygen-carrying capacity of the blood, with some changes at micro-level, is related to the breaking down of the functions of erythrocytes. **If the erythrocyte number is insufficient, then oxygen-carrying capacities will diminish,** as in cases of anemia related to deficiencies of iron, vitamin B12, and folic acid . Thus, anemia should be treated.

Defects in the structure of the erythrocytes also reduce the oxygen-carrying capacity. The blood test we know of as **hemoglobin A1c** is mainly thought to be connected to sugar metabolism disorder. But, there is more. The hemoglobin A1c value increases due to damage to the protein hemoglobin in the erythrocyte, which is caused by the rise of the blood sugar.

Hemoglobin A1c shows the average three-month damage to the erythrocytes.

As the hemoglobin A1c value increases, the erythrocytes' oxygen transport to the tissues diminishes. The oxygen-holding capacity of the "sugared" erythrocytes diminishes. Diabetes-related damage—for instance, the slowdown of wound healing or eye defects—basically arises from both the local damage to the organ due to sugar and the sugared erythrocytes not being able to carry enough oxygen to this organ.

The rise of Hemoglobin A1c can explain hypoxia, the paucity of oxygen in the body at micro-level. **We know that the foods which raise Hemoglobin A1c are floury and sugary foods. In other words, acidifying foods!**

Acidification is a delicate biochemical subject needed to be studied in detail in both the blood and the tissues. The increasing number of studies proves that acidification of tissues and fluids, or the increase of proton charges, is a factor in illnesses. **It can be said that in terms of oxygen, if the pH value of an area shifts to one of acidity, that area will carry less oxygen.**

Owners of aquariums will know that the presence of soluble oxygen in water is related to the aquarium's water being at an alkaline pH so that the fish can breathe. Similar to fish in an aquarium, we are swimming in a huge pool of liquid in our bodies. If the fish get ill in an acidified aquarium, would we change the fish or the water in the aquarium? The same logic is applied to our blood.

The body works to keep the alkaline pH constant in the blood's narrow range. **The buffer systems are in operation 24/7 to remove the plus (+) proton charges that might increase in the blood.** What we need to know is that in an ideal situation, the blood's oxygen-carrying capacity can increase by thirty percent, and in a non-ideal situation diminish by thirty percent. The same situation is also applicable for tissues and other body fluids; when they have the ideal pH, they are able to carry the maximum amount of oxygen.

The function of oxygen—of which if we are deprived for even two to three minutes, we will die—is to reach the mitochondria and provide us with energy. **If there is no oxygen, then there is no energy**. There is death. Decreasing acidity in our diets ensures an increase in the amount of oxygen in our bodies. In other words, when we consume foods containing electrons, it is as though we have taken a breath.

The Brain and Oxygen

The brain forms two percent of the weight of the whole body, but it takes twenty percent of the whole blood-flow for itself. The reason for this is that the brain's cortex, the cause of our evolving, needs a lot of energy. That is why the number of mitochondria in the brain is so high: it has a great need of oxygen for energy.

The difference between primitive primates and

us is the increase in the need for oxygen for the brain tissue. Hence, in primates with undeveloped brains that use little oxygen, the oxygen goes to the muscle. Although their brains are small, their bodies and muscles develop. In humans, however, as evolution progresses, the brain functions increase, and perhaps in the future body functions (e.g., the digestive system) will diminish. Think of the depictions of aliens with huge heads and tiny bodies.

The use of oxygen in the brain is proportional to the blood flow in the brain. The health of the veins must be protected.

We know that the whole body, but the heart and brain in particular, are electrical organs. **Electrical functions need electrons and good fats.** A good brain will develop only if we eat enough of both.

Chapter 6:

IT IS NOT ALL ABOUT FOOD

What Can We Do for Our Quantum Biological Health Apart From Adhering to a Healthy Diet?

Besides food, let's discuss the free and plentiful sources of electrons. As a supplement to our diet, we can contribute to our quantum biological health by replenishing our lives using these sources.

Vitamin G (Grounding)

Diseases do not appear overnight out of nowhere. They are the price we eventually pay for the sins we commit and accumulate against nature every single day. If enough sins are accumulated, illnesses manifest in our bodies. **The first sin we can commit against nature is to lose touch with it.** Most of us spend months without going out into nature, without stepping on soil, and without getting into the sea. Yet, the cost of neglecting nature is great.

First, we have to consider the entire universe and the world, ourselves, and all living organisms as matter with an electromagnetic field. This is because the electromagnetic field inside the earth is positively (+) charged, and the ground and the crust is negatively (-) charged. The earth creates this field by rotating around its own axis. What we are concerned with here is that the earth's surface is negatively (-) charged. **This is because the negative electric charge is caused by electrons, and the earth's crust is a magnificent charging device full of free electrons.** All we need to do to charge ourselves is to be in contact with nature.

Perhaps shoes are the worst invention human beings have ever come up with. Shoes prevent us from capturing the electrons on the surface of the earth, whereas when we step on the damp grass with bare feet, a kind of charging takes place.

When we step on the earth with bare feet, there is a flow of electrons from where there are many to where there are few. We get the free electrons through the soles of our feet when we step on the ground. With their negative (-) charges, these electrons from nature give our positively (+) charged protons, that is the free radicals within us, the negative electrons. They neutralize them.

Stepping on the ground means becoming anti-oxidized!

Stepping on the ground means becoming alkaline!

Direct contact with the earth is therapeutic; it is

what we call "becoming grounded or earthed." The electrons gained from the earth speed up the healing process of illnesses that spread through inflammation. When we step on soil, we benefit from the anti-inflammatory effects of the electrons we acquire. **It is good to walk with bare feet, touch trees and plants, and get into salty seawater to become grounded.** In each case, we are charged with nature's free electrons.

Here we should concentrate on the concept of negative ions. Negative ions are electron-charged ions. The concentration of negative ions is very high in forests, seas, and streams. At home, in the office, and in shopping malls, however, the negative ion concentration is very low. **Many of illnesses in the cities are caused by a scarcity of negative ions.**

In cities, we are eating convenience foods, and so, we are already low on electrons. In addition, when we don't receive negative ions from nature, getting ill becomes inevitable. In some countries, grounding pads of metals such as copper with high electrical conductivity are available in offices. Air conditioners emitting negative ions and alkaline water ionizer machines are used. This practice is still quite rare in some countries. But we are not without remedies. We can opt for the most practical one. **The most practical method is to connect with the earth daily. Twenty minutes is sufficient.**

Protection from Electromagnetic Pollution

Let's remember that we are surrounded by mobile

phones, bluetooth, wi-fi, computers, base stations, and televisions; we live right in the midst of electromagnetic pollution. We know that the earth and our bodies are electromagnetic fields. The negatively charged electromagnetic field transmitted by the earth, us, and other organisms, is healthy. What is unhealthy are the emissions from electronics that create a positive electromagnetic field. The vibrations transmitted by these types of electronics **hack** into the vibrations transmitted by our natural electromagnetic field. As a result of this hacking, we experience problems on a cellular level.

Biophysicists and quantum physicists must cooperate with doctors to establish all of the above, and publish the relevant knowledge in medical literature. A doctor should measure our own electromagnetic fields created by the electric charge on the cell membranes, while a quantum physicist measures the bad electromagnetic field in the environment; when we compare the two, we should be able to see the negativity between them. We should be able to measure the electromagnetic field in our brain when we bring the telephone to our ear. **If you ask any doctor whether mobile phones are harmful, you will not get a proper answer because there is no cooperation in these types of scientific studies.**

The present medical knowledge is fundamentally inadequate for the medical science of the future. Besides biology and biochemistry, every doctor needs to know biophysics and quantum physics. We now know from simple measurements such as the EKG and EEG that the body is a bioelectrical mechanism. Yet, we are not studying this bioelectrical mechanism on the cellular level. The most common cognitive problem encountered among new-generation children is **attention deficit disorder**, and this is perhaps caused by exposure to bad electromagnetic fields at the embryonic stage. Protection from the electromagnetic field will be the main topic of future medicine. For the moment, however, it is important that we try to keep ourselves as far away from these fields as possible.

Sleep

First, we must properly understand the purpose of sleep. Sleep is the state when the body needs to turn back its biological clock. **Sleep is more than rest; it is necessary for repair.** Our consciousness is different during sleep than when we are awake. The brain does this for a purpose. Our brainwaves have different wavelengths during sleep than in the waking hours. These different brainwaves that can be measured easily in sleep laboratories are peculiar to sleep. Without going into detail, it can be said that the purpose of these wavelengths is to give the body the signal to relax.

The purpose of the **parasympathetic system** active during sleep is increased communication and repair between all the cells. Sleep is imperative for this to occur. Even after a day spent on the couch when we haven't become physically tired, we still need to sleep.

We don't sleep because we are physically tired; we sleep to put the body into some sort of "reset" mode.

Our biological clock is called **biorhythm**. Biorhythms are sensitive to light. Yes, once more we are talking about light; that is, sunlight. Sunlight defines the rhythm of nature—all of nature. Everything including the reproduction of animals, flowers, and plants are dependent on this rhythm. There is no escape. And human beings cannot escape it either. Many of the hormones of our endocrine system are released according to this rhythm. The chickens in farms are exposed to light twenty-four hours a day to make them lay more eggs. Because of the light, the endocrine system forces the chicken to continuously lay eggs. This is a simple example illustrating the relationship between light and the endocrine system.

When we stay awake at night because the light is on, we ruin our endocrine system. At night, our endocrine system must continue to produce hormones.

We start producing melatonin, the sleep hormone, at around 11 p.m.; but if we are exposed to light (lamps, mobile phones, television, etc.), the release of the hormone will be prevented.

The hormone melatonin is released when it is dark, and when prevented, the effectiveness of that night's sleep is lost. We are then removed from the

real purpose of sleep, and our repair system will not function.

Our most important hormone after melatonin is the growth hormone. If we go to sleep at the right time, we will acquire a system that is young, thanks to the growth hormone being released. **The growth hormone is not only related to growing but also to repair.**

Eating at night or drinking alcohol will ruin the quality of sleep. The condition called nocturnal hypoglycemia will wake you up in the middle of the night. Late evening meals that include alcohol or are full of carbohydrates disrupt and destroy the quality of your sleep. **The solution is an early evening meal and, of course, to eat alkaline foods.**

The feeling of having had a restful sleep diminishes when the muscles have not relaxed enough. Fibromyalgia, cramps, and restless leg syndrome are, in fact, signs that there is lactic acid in the body's muscles; in other words, it indicates that the cheap Plan B was used to produce energy. The production of energy in the mitochondria declines both through bad carbohydrate- and sugar-ridden nutrition, and when there is oxygen deficiency. Sleep apnea, nose deviation, and a blocked nose due to allergic reactions can also be added to cases of decreasing oxygen.

Waking up tired is very common for all the above-mentioned reasons. **If you do not wake up rested, it is because your mitochondria haven't produced enough energy through the night for repair.** You may be wondering what it is that we can do to achieve good energy during the night, and if this be done through nutrition. First of all, night hunger, the golden rule, is a better choice than eating at night. **Night hunger is the quickest way to recover a healthy sleep pattern.**

- **Go to bed hungry!**

Two things happen during night hunger. The first is **autophagy**. Phagia means eating. Autophagia means to eat one's self; in other words, self-cannibalism. However it may sound, this is good. In the cytoplasm of the cells, there are organelles called **lysosomes**. The antioxidant systems clean up the cell's own trash; while they capture and remove the trash that is still at the proton stage, the lysosomes will eat and destroy the remains of the already-damaged cells, of which the antioxidant systems cannot dispose.

Bacteria, viruses, and other foreign matters are also usually affected by this kind of "eating." Because, they are harmful. The same enzymes will also destroy and wipe out bits of old cells that don't work properly. **In short, autophagy means the dissolving and eradication of damaged cell-parts by enzymes.**

For instance, if you have a tattoo, it will fade in time. The reason for this is that the body's cleaning system is trying to clear away the tattoo. As it can be seen from this example, the body clears away foreign viruses, bacteria, and tattoos, as well as unwanted bits inside the body by "eating" them.

When the autophagy system works correctly, it protects us from all illnesses. Autophagy also protects us from cancer, infections, and brain degeneration. For instance, the body wants to clear away the plaques formed in the brain, in the case of Alzheimer's, with autophagy. Medications activating this system are being developed.

The inexpensive way for us to get rid of the old and renew ourselves through autophagy is to fast. **Intermittent fasting,** or **dinner canceling**, are examples of fasting methods. Another method to increase autophagy is moderate exercise. A ketogenic diet of good fat and plentiful vegetables, no carbohydrates, and a minimum of proteins also aids autophagy.

One of the purposes of sleep is to give the body fasting time and thereby give autophagy an opportunity. This is due to some sort of **ketosis** happening during the night. Another way to put it is that at night we burn only fat because we are hungry, and this increases cell renewal.

In anti-aging studies, the method proven to prolong life the most is the "eat-less method." When less is eaten, the **long-life genes** in the body, the **sirtuin genes**, are activated. In my opinion, it is **"what"** is eaten that is important rather than eating "less." The reason for this is that, similar to the eat-less model, there are foodstuffs that activate the sirtuin genes. **Let me be more specific: the main nutrients that activate the** longevity gene are purple fruits and vegetables.

Fasting in the evening ensures improvements not only on the cellular level but also on our blood tests. **All we need to do is have our evening meals as early as 5 p.m.** Recovery from illnesses such as insulin resistance, fatty liver disease, weight problems, and illnesses that progress due to inflammations, as well as many other problems can easily be attained by implementing this method. Even psychological recovery is possible through evening-fasting. Your sleep will be better as it will not be interrupted by **nocturnal hypoglycaemia** in the middle of the night after a late meal of bad carbohydrates, for instance. A good night's sleep leads to a better mental state the following day.

Something else that happens when you fast is that your **dopamine receptors** become active. Dopamine provides a *joie de vivre* as this hormone is related to pleasure. When the dopamine receptors have become sensitive after fasting, we enjoy the next meal even more. Indeed, the first mouthful of food after a fast is quite special. This is due to the sensitized dopamine receptors. Let me reiterate that dopamine isn't related to appetite but to pleasure. In fact, dopamine ensures quick satisfaction, and it controls the appetite. If there is enough dopamine, our pangs of hunger diminish. **Love also increases dopamine. When we are in love, we don't feel hungry.**

Chapter 7:

METHODS TO FORTIFY THE BODY

Detox: Toxin-Clearance Support

The ability to clear the toxins, the metabolic waste, is related to a person's health as well as to the consumption of the right foods. We know that there is waste that needs to be expelled even with the ideal choice of food. The waste we obtain from the environment is also added to normal metabolic waste; substances polluting the air such as heavy metals, exhaust and cigarettes, chemicals and preservatives in all kinds of food and cosmetics, plastics, drugs, microbial substances, alcohol, and so on—we can make this list much longer. **All these need to be expelled from the body.**

The most important organ for detoxification is the liver. The liver filters the blood, forms bile, and **detoxifies** through detox systems—namely, phase 1 and phase 2. The liver filters two liters of blood per minute. It cleans the body's natural waste, which is formed at the end of all the blood's metabolic processes and, which needs to be expelled daily. In addition to this, it also cleans the chemicals, preservatives, and pesticides we digest with food and that pass to the blood. If the intestinal permeability has been upset, the bacteria and toxins that seep in through the intestine create antigens and antibody complexes, which are a burden on the immune system. The liver is responsible for clearing away these as well.

In using phase 1 and phase 2 detoxification stages, the liver makes the toxins non-toxic and removes them from the body. In order for the fat-soluble toxins to be removed, they have to be made water-soluble. This is the work of the liver. When the toxins become water-soluble, they are either expelled with bile from the intestines as feces, or from the kidneys as urine.

The liver produces approximately one liter of bile a day. The production of bile is necessary for the many poisonous substances that have been detoxed in the liver to be effectively removed from the body. So that removal by bile is complete, when the toxins in the bile are discharged into the intestine, there have to be food fibers in the intestine to hold them there. **Constipation, which may cause reabsorption of the bile toxins, also needs to avoided.**

Now let's take a look at the phases of liver detox. First of all, there is phase 1. The problem with phase 1 is that these toxic substances have to be sent subsequently to phase 2 for cleaning. **These two phases complement one another.** However, if the second-phase detox in the liver doesn't function well, then intermediate metabolites form; unfortunately, these are far more dangerous than the original substances.

In the first phase in the liver, excess hormones in the body as well as medications and chemicals are detoxified. Examples of these hormones are as follows: histamine, the cause of allergic reactions; estrogen, which increases fibroids and cysts; cortisol, which emerges with stress; and testosterone, which triggers prostate cancer. Anything over the daily required amount is detoxed.

There is a system identified as **cytochrome P450** that enables phase 1 detox. Every enzyme, between fifty and a hundred, detoxes a different chemical substance. In some individuals, the detox system in phase 1 is genetically slow. The easiest method in understanding this is to discover how the person detoxifies coffee.

- When coffee keeps you awake, it is an indication that coffee is detoxified late from your blood and liver.

The dangerous intermediate metabolites formed during the passage from phase 1 to phase 2 are, in fact, **free radicals**. If there are not enough antioxidant substances in the liver to prevent these free radicals, it will cause damage to the liver. It is for this reason that **glutathione**, the most important antioxidant of them all, is in the liver.

However, if there are many toxins in phase 1, and phase 2 functions slowly, the glutathione, which removes the free radicals, will run out. But glutathione is also essential for cleanup in phase 2. As with phase 1, phase 2 can also be slow in some people. Ultimately, poisonous intermediate products will still remain. For this, "**methylation**, **sulfation**, and **acetylation**" chemical detox-methods are used in cleaning of the liver in phase 2.

In simple terms, the foods and supplements below must be increased to support the liver's detox-phases:

- Foods Containing Sulphur

One of the methods the liver uses for detoxification is sulfation. The liver uses sulfation on some toxins, thereby making them harmless. This group has special importance in detoxification because of the sulphur they contain. Sulphur increases glutathione, the most important substance for detoxification.

- kale

- broccoli

- brussel sprouts

- cauliflower

- garlic

- onions

- Artichoke—The silibinin it contains is a powerful liver supplement.

- Turmeric—It is a protectant, powerful antioxidant, and anti-inflammatory for the liver's mitochondria. As a nutrient, it is the most effective antitumor agent.

- Green Tea—It is a great antioxidant.

Vitamin Supplements

- The vitamin B group—in particular, B6, B12, and folic acid

- Vitamin C—it is an antioxidant that helps glutathione to be repeatedly used.

- Vitamin D

- DIM and I3C (diindolylmethane and indole-3-carbinol)—these are similar substances. They have a broccoli-like content. They are particularly important in protection against breast cancer. They detoxify surplus estrogen.

- Selenium—It is a substance that assists glutathione in detoxification. Selenium deficiency is generally widespread in Turkey and Europe as there is little selenium in the soil. It is particularly useful in the removal of heavy metals.

Methylation Donors

Methylation is one of the methods used in detoxifying the liver. Slowness of methylation is genetically widespread in people in some countries; for instance, in Turkey. These supplements are suggested to improve the strength of methylation.

- SAMe (S-Adenosylmethionine)
- N-acetylcysteine (NAC)
- Methylfolate
- Methyl B12
- TMG (Trimethylglycine)

In phase 2 of cleansing the liver, apart from sulfation and methylation I mentioned above, the chemical detox methods **acetylation** and **glucuronidation** are used. However, nutrients that also support both phases in every way are the plant foods and supplements listed above.

Besides the liver, the kidneys, intestine, and skin are our other major systems of detoxification. **The proper functioning of these macrosystems again depends on the proper functioning of the mitochondria**. The necessary energy for cleaning comes from the mitochondria. If the mitochondria of these organs produce enough energy, detoxification will be easier. We should have the right nutrients for energy to be sufficient. The right nutrients are the same foods we have mentioned throughout this book.

In brief, eating alkaline foods, all raw fruits and vegetables, spices, good vegetable fats with their antioxidants (their electrons) support detoxification.

Let's briefly sum up how we can assist the detoxification process of our bodies:

- eating raw fruits and vegetables

- drinking plenty of water

- sweating in heat and saunas—especially infrared saunas

- lymph massage

- bouncing on trampolines

- increasing probiotic foods

- exercise

- avoiding constipation

- grounding

- sleeping well

However, we must remember that whatever process is carried out in the body—this includes removing toxins, it all starts inside the mitochondrion.

Therefore, in order to provide energy for all the metabolism-related processes in the body, we must also support the removal of toxins as well as supporting our mitochondria.

Chapter 8:

THOSE WHO VALUE THEIR LIFE PROTECT THEIR MITOCHONDRIA

Charging the Mitochondria

For vitality, we need energy. Luckily, we have millions of energy-batteries. These mitochondria-batteries keep us constantly charged. Let's take a look at how we can increase their charges while the mitochondria charge us.

Oxygen is the first and foremost requirement!

As living organisms that need to breathe, we must increase the conduction of oxygen to the mitochondria. The health of our lungs is obviously very important for our breathing capacity to increase. I leave it up to you to think about and deal with the major factors that lower oxygen levels such as illnesses caused by allergies, the holding of breath for psychological reasons, nasal problems, sleep apnea, sleep disorders, and smoking.

But even if we get the proper, sufficient breath at micro level, how can we increase the transportation of oxygen to its target? When the breath enters the body from the lungs, it is transported by the blood and the erythrocytes in the blood. **This means that, first of all, the blood vessels need to be sound.** Their volume should not be reduced by plaque or hardening of the arteries. **For the fluidity of blood to be good**, it is imperative that oxygen is transported to the cells and mitochondria of the organs furthest away in the body.

High blood sugar levels, a cause of diminishing fluidity of the blood, should be regulated. Because when the sugar level is high, the capacity of the hemoglobin in the erythrocytes to carry oxygen decreases. We should understand that many complaints of diabetic patients, such as wounds not healing, cataracts, and kidney diseases are linked to the fact that blood with a high glucose content does not carry oxygen sufficiently. **Diabetes is a type of asphyxiation at a micro level**.

We know that the blood's ideal pH is between 7.35 and 7.45. This does not change. But if the pH falls by just 0.1, the blood's capacity to carry oxygen decreases by thirty percent. **In other words, if we stick to an ideal diet and lifestyle, we breathe one-third more than people who have chosen a bad lifestyle.**

It is not only blood; our entire body is actually a liquid pool. One could say that we actually live in an aquarium. All our cells are full of liquid. The mitochondria inside them are also full of liquid. All this liquid has an ideal pH balance. The mitochondrial matrix of a pH level between 8 and 8.5 makes it the most alkaline part of the cell. The reason for this is the electron transport chain, where energy is produced.

Another name for the electron transport chain is the **respiratory chain**. This is the place where the oxygen that comes from breathing is used. If the pH of the respiratory chain has remained highly alkaline, the rate at which this place meets with oxygen increases— as it is with alkaline blood. The really big energy-prize to be gained from nutrition is this electron transport chain. So how do we keep it alkaline?

Remember that to be alkaline, a surplus negative (-) charge has to be secured. The mitochondrial matrix is generally the highest negatively (-) charged and lowest positively (+) charged part of the body. This is because the protons that form the positive (+) charges are pumped out of there by the energy of the electron transport chain. The energy for this pump comes from the food's electrons.

- The conclusion is that eating plenty of electrons equals to the ability to use plenty of oxygen.
- When we eat plant-based foods, we actually eat oxygen.
- To eat plant-based foods means to breathe.

In order to increase the amount of oxygen carried by the

blood, there must be a sufficient number of erythrocytes. **As there are not enough erythrocytes in anemia, we cannot get enough oxygen**. The production of oxygen-derived energy decreases, and we feel tired. The most typical anemia is caused by a lack of folic acid, B12, and iron. In these cases, B12, folate, and iron supplements should be taken as advised by a doctor.

Omega-3 supplements are beneficial for increasing the fluidity of the blood in the blood vessels. The omega-3 fatty acids are the fatty acids found on the erythrocyte cell membranes. Their deficiency changes the voltage on the cell membranes of the erythrocytes. The erythrocytes—that normally push one another— attract one another when the voltage changes and they cluster. If they cluster, the fluidity of the blood decreases.

Using supplements containing **ginkgo biloba** also increases the oxygen that is carried to the cells. This is why supplements containing ginkgo are used for memory loss and brain-related problems.

Low blood pressure should also be viewed with as a problem. Many women have low blood pressure of around 80/50 rather than 120/80. Low blood pressure indicates that when the heart pumps blood, it is not being exerted, and the blood vessels in front of the heart are soft. This softness is related to the collagen structure of the blood vessels. It is one advantage of the female hormone estrogen that keeps the skin pliant. **However,**

the low blood pressure may mean that the blood does not reach the extremities of the body. Sudden blackouts when standing up, dizziness, cold—and pale—hands and feet as well as easy bruising in cold weather are indicative of low blood pressure. **Where the blood doesn't travel, oxygen will not travel, either.**

Blood pressure can be increased a unit by making **SOLE (a mixture of sea salt and water)** and using it daily, which may lessen relevant symptoms. Using salt is also important because we need the electrolytes inside it. The electrical performance of a liquid without any minerals is low, while minerals such as salt increase electrical conductivity.

Exercise is also important for the blood to circulate throughout the body. Slow tempo exercises have a beneficial effect on blood pressure. They help the blood and oxygen circulate everywhere. That is the purpose of sports.

Fats are also a better energy source than sugar for obtaining energy through oxygen. Since we know that the mitochondria are the only place where fat can be burned, the way to lose weight, or rather to use our own fat as fuel, is through healthy and sufficiently oxygenated mitochondria.

External Supplements to Repair Mitochondria

In order to increase the functions of our mitochondria, we can also take enzymes and cofactors of the internal biochemical activities as external support. What are they? Let's take a closer look.

CoQ10 (Coenzyme Q10)

This is the mitochondria's main support. CoQ10 is generally known to be recommended for heart disease. The heart's need for energy means that it has a lot of mitochondria. CoQ10 helps increase the energy of the heart. The triad that consists of the heart, muscles, and brain likes to use fat for these organs' needs for high energy. They especially prefer medium- and short-chain fats. When it comes to burning fat, because the mitochondria are involved, the mitochondria in the organs that need high energy use more CoQ10.

CoQ10 is a substance from the ETS chain, which carries the electrons from one area to another in the ETS system. Since CoQ10 is the electron-carrier in this system, it creates enough energy to remove the protons from the area. **In other words, CoQ10 is a kind of antioxidant that protects the mitochondria. It synthesizes in the body but is also found in food**. It is a substance that dissolves in fat. This is why it is also found on the membranes.

Foods from which CoQ10 can be obtained:

- soy
- soybeans
- fish

- hazelnuts

- broccoli

- oranges

- eggs

- liver

- cauliflower

- chicken

- sweet potatoes

- butter

- avocado

- apples

- black pepper

- olive oil

- PQQ (pyrroloquinoline quinone)

This is a substance similar to CoQ10. It is known as the antioxidant within the mitochondria. It increases the energy and self-repair of the mitochondria. **The greatest source is dark chocolate and unprocessed cocoa.**

L-Carnitine

This secures the conveyance of long-chain fats from the

cytoplasm to the mitochondria, and as a result, more energy is obtained from fats. Without L-carnitine, long-chain fats cannot be burned but short- and medium-chain fats can. The acetyl L-carnitine version is more effective. **Lamb is a rich natural source of L-carnitine. Fish, poultry, asparagus, avocado, and wheat are among foods that also contain L-carnitine.**

D-Ribose

This is a type of sugar that is the fastest in converting to energy in the mitochondria. It is used to increase the performance of athletes, to treat congestive heart failure, muscle weakness, fibromyalgia, and some forms of anemia.

Selenium

This is the cofactor of the antioxidant system inside the mitochondria. It also retains the heavy metals inside the mitochondria. It increases glutathione and balances the thyroid hormones.

Alpha Lipoic Acid

This is an antioxidant that dissolves both in fat and in liquid. It is the antioxidant in the mitochondrial membrane (fat) and the cell cytoplasm (water). It ensures the repeated use of other antioxidants (vitamin E and vitamin C). **The R-alpha lipoic acid** version is more effective.

Other oral supplements

Other recommended vitamin supplements that also ensure the health of the mitochondria are:

- glutathione precursors (NAC, SAMe, cysteine, methyl-B12, methylfolate)

- magnesium

- vitamin B1

- vitamin B6

Others supporting the mitochondrial membrane apart from omega-3:

- phosphatidylserine

- phosphatidylcholine

- cardiolipin

- ginkgo biloba—that increases oxygen going to the mitochondria

- concentrated plant supplements that contain antioxidants—resveratrol, polyphenol, pycnogenol, and silymarin.

Apart from these oral supplements there are also cocktails providing support at the most advanced level which are administered intravenously and contain special antioxidant vitamins for the mitochondria.

Chapter 9:

Quantum Communication

In the body, there is a very fast communication network between all cells. This communication happens through electrons, photons, and electromagnetic fields that conform to the laws of quantum physics.

If quantum physics seems new and confusing, we can continue to understand this communication with classical physics. We know that we are electrical living organisms. Methods such as EEG and EKG show that we have an electrical communication network. So how does it happen?

Again, as you can guess, electrons are in play. The flow of electrons on a conductor from where they are concentrated to where they are few is called a **direct current circuit (DC)**. Electrons exit from the electron transport chain in this way. Here, a DC is formed. The electrical flow in the whole human body is a DC. The electrical current we use in our homes, however, is called an **alternating current (AC)**.

We now know that if there are plenty of electrons, or if the structure of the conductor providing their current is good, the electric voltage is ideal. Electrons flow in the mitochondrion's inner membrane. In other words, the conductor is this membrane.

Conductivity is provided by the fats on these membranes. We also know how important the membrane is. **If the membrane is bad, energy will decrease. If there is no energy, there is no work, and the system becomes nonoperational**. If the fats in the membranes are damaged by free radicals, they will oxidize, and free radical damage called lipid peroxidation will occur.

Lipid peroxidation, besides appearing in every illness, is observed more in cardiovascular diseases. The oxidization of LDL (bad cholesterol) forms the basis of cardiovascular diseases. The oxidization of LDL means LDL is being attacked by free radicals. It is an indication that there is little antioxidant protection in the veins. In heart and vascular diseases, the sources of antioxidants—that is, foods containing electrons— must immediately be increased.

The decrease of the membranes' electrical conductivity, which consequently leads to the decrease of their voltage, will also decrease the communication between cells. Yet all cells communicate with one another instantly, faster than the speed of electricity. **Deceleration in this communication speed can manifest itself in the simplest terms as slowed-down reflexes or remembering something later.**

This communication speed is very important on a micro level. The electrical environment on the cell membrane creates an **electromagnetic field (EMF)**. Therefore, the cells actually communicate between themselves through this EMF. What is more, the EMF emitted by the cells is stronger in places where electrical energy is plentiful in the body. Considering that the heart and brain use the most energy and the most oxygen and have the most mitochondria, the strongest EMF is found in these areas. This broad EMF field can interact with other EMF fields outside the body.

The world's EMF field is in harmony with living organisms, including us. For instance, birds find direction with this EMF. However, the EMF field created by technological devices is not in harmony with animate beings. The electromagnetic field emitted by mobile phones, computers, televisions, shopping malls, Wi-Fi, and electrical appliances such as hairdryers is contrary to our EMF and has a detrimental effect on our EMF—that is, our conductivity.

Even humans have different EMFs between them. When you embrace someone who is fond of you, their EMF field mixes with yours. **Indeed, if some people make you feel good, it is due to the influence of their**

EMF. When you hug a person who has plenty of electrons, you will take electrons from them if you have only a few. That is why it makes one feel good to hug babies, animals, and trees.

Quantum Brain

For a long time, the subject of cholesterol, research into veins, the health of organs—the heart, kidneys, liver, etc.— have received priority in medicine. This is due to fact that diseases and symptoms of these organs emerge more quickly than the symptoms caused by brains eventually wearing out.

Yet, now we know that our most valuable asset is the brain, or rather the mitochondria inside our brain.

Our intelligence, our skills, our memory, and even our feelings and the way we perceive events are related to the health of our brain cells. The hypothesis which states that we came into the world with a certain brain-function capacity and that it cannot be increased is old and mistaken. The new knowledge is that the brain is a changing, developing organ that can restructure itself in new forms. This restructuring called **brain plasticity** is the key topic in modern neurology.

Plasticity refers to brain cells increasing their elasticity, which occurs when they gain new skills. What the brain can do is a hundred percent related to how we feed it. "Feeding the brain" is now a true expression in the strictest sense. It has also been acknowledged that the brain is a computer. **In conclusion, the brain is, in fact, not only a biological structure but a type of quantum biological computer.**

For the quantum biology of the brain, one needs to obviously look at its atoms. The nerve cells in the brain are neurons. Neurons communicate with one another with special receptors and special chemicals called **neurotransmitters**. An electrical flow is generated in the networks between the neurons. For instance, an EEG measurement shows us the electrical current in the brain.

Electrical signal transmission in the brain occurs with negatively charged electrons moving along through the nerve cells. Here, the amount of electricity is made up from the difference in voltage between the inside and outside of the brain cells' membrane. The inside of the cell is negatively charged while the outside is positively charged. The difference in a single cell creates a difference in voltage of up to one percent of one volt. Although it does not seem much, let's not forget that the cell membranes are just a few nanometers thick. In other words, this difference is a tiny distance. **When we apply it to meters, the electrical difference that emerges is one million volts per meter.** This is exactly like the energy level needed to create a spark similar to the spark needed to ignite the fuel in the spark plugs of your car.

What you should realize here is that we always need this difference in voltage to enable transmission from the brain to the body. The inside of properly functioning brain- and nerve-system cells is negatively (-) charged; that is, there are more electrons, and their pH is alkaline. **It is important to know how we can assist the brain by ensuring this with food. The measures I have mentioned throughout this book are necessary to provide maximum brain capacity.**

As the brain ages, the cerebral cortex—which has taken us to the top step in the stairs of evolution—is the last to age. It is in this place that memory and analytical thought is located. Losses of nerve cells occur more in the lower parts, which are relatively less active in daily life. However, damage to sections of memory and thought capacity eventually occur with time.

As a result of brain scans, it is believed that the blood traveling to the brain tissue—the grey matter—begins to decrease around age fifty for the following reason: older brains have much more difficulty in generating energy while registering information. This is due to the functions of the mitochondria diminishing with aging, in other words, the decrease in energy production.

Mitochondria produce energy in the brain cells as they do in every cell. So, of course, free radical damage accumulates. **This is why diseases such as Alzheimer's, Parkinson's, and dementia generally emerge in old age.** Even if we are not ill, the protection of our intellectual capacity depends on minimizing the production of free radicals. Foods consisting of antioxidants, or electrons, can also recycle the damage in the brain, as they can in other organs.

It is never too late to begin to protect your brain; it is never too early to protect your brain!

In light of this, what to do in terms of diet is simple. You should have memorized it by now: increase foods containing electrons!

The brain uses most of the glucose in the blood. However, if the source of the glucose is bad carbohydrates, then the production of free radicals will increase. By bad carbohydrates, I mean foods that are floury, sugary, and that do not contain the sun's energy or electrons as they have been processed. **When they have absorbed the sunlight with photosynthesis and have sprouted, grains such as barley and wheat contain more electrons and are much more superior to foods that have been processed in a factory.**

Let's not forget that most chemicals related to emotion are secreted from the brain. For our emotion-hormones—**also know as serotonin and dopamine— to function well, the cell membrane must be pliable and thin**. If the membranes are thick, a person will feel the need for a higher dose of the hormone to be satisfied. The amounts of hormones serotonin (happiness) or dopamine (*joie de vivre*) have to be increased in order for us to feel positive.

This is why current lifestyles and diet choices—the cause of the hardening of the brain cell membranes—

make us unhappy. Things that used to easily make us happy no longer please us. If you are someone who easily becomes happy, you should keep in mind that your brain membranes are still quite good.

In that case, we can say that omega-3, fish, nuts (e.g., walnuts and almonds), seed oils, spices, and plants each function as an antidepressant. Being outdoors and solving our breathing problems similarly work as antidepressants.

Furthermore, like other cells, the outer membranes of the brain cells should be very fatty. Sixty percent of the brain cells is fat. If we keep the abundance of unsaturated fat in the membranes, the electrons there will increase the vibration and facilitate the electrical current in the membranes. There is an electromagnetic field in every place where electricity flows.

The brain's electromagnetic field is a quantum biological event. All the cells in the brain function with **instant communication** without losing so much as a second. This is called **coherence** in the brain. Coherence can be increased or decreased. A decrease is not a desirable situation; it slows down the brain functions.

Meditation is when coherence increases the most. Meditation performs a kind of tuning, and enables all the cell membranes to be on the same wavelength. It is right here that the brain can be used with maximum capacity. Creativity and concentration can similarly be ensured with the

increase of coherence in the brain.

The moment the mind focuses on a thought—when coherence between the brain cells is at its maximum—actually explains the case of the **"secret"** in new age approaches. Let's bear in mind the brain's holographic structure, and that it is a quantum computer.

The holographic brain means that every cell of the brain has all the information at the same time. When we concentrate and focus on a thought in the frontal lobe, the cortex, we create that thought holographically in the brain. **Just like the light of a laser focusing on a single spot, concentrated thinking focuses the thought on the brain's frontal lobe.** The creation of this state of concentration occurs with the electrical firing between neurons. For instance, if you wish to think of a banana, thousands of neurons fire at the same moment. Electricity flows amongst them and draws a holographic, three dimensional yellow banana on your frontal lobe.

This electrical current between neurons creates an electromagnetic field belonging to this thought around the brain. Because the intensity of thought is proportionate to the power of electrical firing, high concentration creates a higher electromagnetic field. What I have explained so far is medical. **However, with quantum physics coming into play, we can add this: the electromagnetic field created by thought attracts other electromagnetic fields compatible with itself.**

If we were to compare this to broadcasting from a radio station, we would hear frequencies compatible with the transmission frequencies we are using. Therefore, expressions such as the "quantum law of attraction" in new age tenets try to explain this matter technically.

For good, strong electromagnetic fields, we see that cell-to-cell coherence in the brain has to be high. **Providing the ideal biochemical conditions for brain cells to supply this is possible by following the guidelines on diet and lifestyle in this book.**

With quantum physics, even the concept of time is different from before. We now know that time is not linear but that we perceive it as such. We create the seeds of events of the future with electromagnetic fields belonging to our thoughts of a given moment. **In that case, let's keep this powerful quantum computer of ours at its best performance, so that the electricity and electromagnetic field it transmits can be more powerful.** Accordingly, we should be able to approach events that are compatible with our own thought-electricity from the **"alternative future probability pool."**

Let's conclude that quantum eating is imperative for a happy, healthy brain and a bright future!

Epilogue

- ❖ What creates aging differences between people?

- ❖ Why do some people get less ill than others?

- ❖ Why do some of us feel tired and weary while some of us are energetic?

- ❖ While hundreds of diseases of different names have been identified, do they each have different causes?

- ❖ Are the cells in the organs which have those diseases different from each other?

- ❖ Should one consult a different physician for each disease?

- ❖ In order to live a healthy and long life without illness, which doctor, or who, should we consult about which organ?

- ❖ The medicine of the future will merely be to prevent initial damage.

- ❖ In the future, physicians will not be diagnosing diseases.

Consequently, there will no longer be such a thing as curing diseases. Medicine, biophysics, biomedicine, quantum physics, and electronics will be intertwined, and the system faults will be dealt with at micro and molecular levels. There will be a greater need for quantum biologists than for surgeons.

These are not exaggerations, they just need broader thinking. Since we accept that we are biological creatures, we must stop ignoring the biology of our smallest units—the cells, and the organelles inside them. The secret that makes the human being a special living species is hidden in the system inside these cells. The cells' own inner processes, energy production, intercellular communication, the cell systems' functioning as a whole, the cells being synchronized with the earth, sun, and universe occur entirely according to the rules of quantum biology. These are subatomic events that seem strange to us.

Subatomic little particles (not just electrons and protons but quarks, tachyons, etc.) and information about their effects on health and vitality will in time be a source of amazement. Throughout this book, I have only attempted to clarify matters at the cell and mitochondria levels—the deepest points to which we can go down. **If we can understand even this much, we can establish the link between our health and getting ill.**

Let's now summarize what we have discussed throughout this book.

✓ Fruit and vegetables should be consumed raw, with their skins, and organic (if possible).

✓ Seeds—especially fatty seeds—should be consumed.

✓ Nuts should be consumed raw and soaked in water.

✓ Pulses should be consumed either germinated or boiled.

✓ The consumption of high-fat vegetables, such as avocados, coconuts, and olives should be increased.

✓ We should remember that the other good fats are fish, butter, krill, and astaxanthin.

✓ Every mouthful of food should be well-chewed.

✓ Water should be drunk sufficiently.

✓ Attention should be paid to oxygen and breathing.

✓ Daily contact should be made with the earth

✓ Daily contact should also be made with the sun for vitamin D.

✓ Sleep performance should be enhanced.

✓ Evening fasting, dinner canceling, and intermittent fasting should be frequently adopted to support autophagy.

✓ Light exercise such as bouncing on trampolines, yoga, and walking should be undertaken.

✓ Animal proteins should be consumed at a minimum. One gram per kilogram is enough. Fish, eggs, turkey, organic red meat, cheese curd, bone broth, trotter soup, and liver are good proteins that come to mind.

✓ Intestinal health should be maintained with probiotics and fiber support.

Now, let me make my last comment…

Even if you were not interested in reading this book for your health, you can support your efforts to create the future you want with your diet and lifestyle through what you have learned.

Wishing you all the best for the future…

I thank you for the patience you have shown in reading this book, which is so full of technical details.

Sincerely yours,

Dr. Ayşegül Çoruhlu

January 2017

Bonus:

On the one hand, poets and writers keep talking about love in their works; one the other hand, love has a medical biochemistry. To desire someone, to fall in love, and to be faithful, or unfaithful, are all related to our hormones.

Where is the secret of ever-lasting love? Why do we become attached to certain people and readily abandon others?

The answer is hidden in the love hormone oxytocin.

Just like "the happiness hormone" serotonin and the hormone dopamine—that makes people look for excitement—oxytocin directs our feelings. Generally, oxytocin is a hormone released from our mothers during birth and suckling, ensuring the mother's unconditional bond with her child. However, when it is a question of love, oxytocin is active in both women and men. In women, it emerges after orgasm. Nature has found this perfect method for attachment to a partner. It is the reason that women are more successful in mating for life. Oxytocin is increased after every orgasm, and an attachment to the partner is formed.

In men, oxytocin develops in a similar way. Sex and contact, such as embracing and stroking, brings out oxytocin in men as well. As long as there is oxytocin, both sides tend to trust each other and be faithful to one another. Indeed, in many publications you have likely come across oxytocin being referred to as "the fidelity hormone" as well as "the love hormone."

Unfortunately, not everyone may have the same amount of oxytocin. Oxytocin deficiency in men may create a feeling of dissatisfaction and "wanting to leave." If what I claim appears to be nonsense, I may be able to persuade you with this: oxytocin has such a powerful tension-reducing and love-arousing side to it that in order to suppress fights in prisons in the United States, oxytocin was sprayed in the noses of the prisoners as an experiment and found to be successful. The *Liquid Trust* hormone is even for sale there.

Now, what happens if oxytocin is low in a man or woman? There is an increase in relationships connected with the hormone dopamine—the opposite of oxytocin, the hormone of commitment and love. In other words, people choose exciting relationships—which fuel the pleasure and reward system and are the equivalent to a kind of addiction, but are basically difficult to tolerate emotionally for a long period of time. In relationships based on dopamine, people find themselves running in pursuit of short-lasting gratification, like being addicted to cigarettes or craving something sweet, despite the damage.

Contrarily, when oxytocin is present, not only do we feel ourselves in a secure, loving relationship but we also have the bonus of this hormone's other physically healing aspects.

Oxytocin does the following:

- increases immunity
- is an anti-inflammatory
- delays cell aging
- speeds up the process of wound healing
- reduces allergic reactions
- normalizes appetite
- deepens sleep
- relieves pain

I don't know whether you attach importance to all these benefits of oxytocin or to the fact that it is "the fidelity hormone"; but if you are asking how we can increase oxytocin, again, it is all about healthy alkaline eating.

1. Since the cells where oxytocin is secreted and where it has an impact are in the brain, the most important step to take is to increase the response of our cells in the brain to this hormone. And here, the sole rule is through "oiling" the outer membranes of the brain cells. By this I mean omega-3 fatty acids. The more the brain cell membranes contain omega-3 derived fats, the better the situation hormonally. Krill oil and astaxanthin are important at this juncture.

2. The notion that sugar is good for brain cells is not quite correct. Rather than sugar, the brain needs as I have stated, omega-3 and other good fats, fatty seeds (black cumin, linseed, etc.) and fatty nuts (almonds, walnuts, etc.). These fats increase the brain cells' sensitivity to all kinds of hormones, including oxytocin.

3. All the advice on diet (with vegetables, fruits, alkaline water, spices, seeds, fish, etc.), breathing good oxygen, sleeping well, and avoiding processed foods—the basis of alkaline living—will have long lasting benefits, as well as serving to ensure fidelity in love!

Whether you believe it or not, what we call emotion is basically created by the hormones in the brain. If the hormones are changed, emotion can be changed. The opposite is more difficult, however. The way to regulate the hormones is by getting the cells into shape one by one, and this is possible with alkaline eating and alkaline living.

Made in the USA
Las Vegas, NV
25 October 2023